Embracing

Menopause Naturally

By

Calvin M. Duncan

Table of Contents

Chapter One

Introduction

Understanding Menopause

Menopause is a natural biological process that marks the end of a woman's reproductive years. It typically occurs in women between the ages of 45 and 55, although it can happen earlier or later for some individuals. Menopause is characterized by the cessation of menstruation and a decrease in the production of hormones like estrogen and progesterone. This transition can bring about various physical and emotional changes in women, which can have significant impacts on their overall well-being.

To better understand menopause, it is essential to delve into its stages and symptoms. Menopause is typically divided into three stages: perimenopause, menopause, and postmenopause. Perimenopause refers to the period leading up to menopause when hormonal fluctuations begin to occur. Women may experience irregular menstrual cycles, hot flashes, night sweats, mood swings, and sleep disturbances during this stage. Menopause itself is defined as the point when a woman has not had a menstrual period for twelve consecutive months. Finally, postmenopause refers to the years following menopause, during which women may continue to experience symptoms but at a reduced intensity.

The most well-known symptom of menopause is hot flashes. These sudden sensations of heat can cause sweating, flushing, and an elevated heart rate. Hot flashes can be disruptive to a woman's daily life, affecting her sleep quality and overall comfort. Additionally, menopause can lead to vaginal dryness, which can cause discomfort during intercourse and increase the risk of urinary tract infections. Other common symptoms include mood swings, irritability, fatigue, weight gain, decreased libido, and changes in skin and hair texture.

The physical changes associated with menopause are primarily due to the decline in estrogen levels. Estrogen plays a crucial role in maintaining bone density, so its reduction can lead to an increased risk of osteoporosis. Women going through menopause should prioritize bone health through regular exercise, a balanced diet rich in calcium and vitamin D, and, in some cases, hormone replacement therapy (HRT). Estrogen also affects the cardiovascular system, and its decline can contribute to an increased risk of heart disease and stroke. Therefore, it is essential for women to adopt heart-healthy lifestyle habits, such as regular exercise, a healthy diet, and avoiding smoking and excessive alcohol consumption.

While menopause is a natural process, it can still have a significant impact on a woman's mental health. The hormonal fluctuations during perimenopause and menopause can lead to mood swings, irritability, anxiety, and even depression. It is crucial for women to seek support from healthcare professionals, friends, and family members during this time. Psychotherapy and

counseling can be beneficial for managing the emotional challenges associated with menopause. Additionally, maintaining a healthy lifestyle through regular exercise, a balanced diet, and stress management techniques like meditation or yoga can help alleviate some of the emotional symptoms.

Understanding menopause also involves recognizing that it is not a one-size-fits-all experience. Each woman may experience different symptoms and have varying degrees of intensity. Some women may transition through menopause with minimal disruption to their daily lives, while others may struggle with severe symptoms that require medical intervention. It is important for women to listen to their bodies and seek appropriate medical care if needed.

In recent years, there has been an increasing focus on alternative treatments for menopause symptoms. Some women turn to herbal supplements like black cohosh or evening primrose oil, while others explore acupuncture or yoga. While these approaches may provide relief for some women, it is important to consult with a healthcare professional before starting any alternative treatment to ensure safety and effectiveness.

In conclusion, menopause is a natural and inevitable phase in a woman's life that marks the end of her reproductive years. It brings about various physical and emotional changes due to hormonal fluctuations. Understanding the stages and symptoms of menopause is crucial for women to navigate this transition with greater ease. Seeking support from healthcare professionals, adopting a healthy lifestyle, and exploring alternative treatments can all contribute to a smoother menopausal experience. With the right knowledge and support, women can embrace menopause as a natural part of life's journey.

Importance of a Natural Approach

The importance of a natural approach to menopause cannot be overstated. Menopause is a natural biological process that every woman will go through at some point in her life. It is not a disease or a condition that needs to be treated, but rather a transition that should be embraced and understood.

One of the primary reasons why a natural approach is important is because it allows women to honor and respect their bodies. Menopause is a natural part of the aging process, and it signifies the end of a woman's reproductive years. By embracing this transition and viewing it as a normal part of life, women can develop a healthier relationship with their bodies and gain a deeper understanding of themselves.

A natural approach to menopause also promotes overall well-being. Menopause can bring about various physical and emotional changes, and it is important for women to prioritize their health during this time. By adopting a natural approach, women can focus on maintaining a healthy lifestyle, which includes regular exercise, a balanced diet, stress management techniques, and self-care practices.

Regular exercise is crucial during menopause as it can help alleviate symptoms such as hot flashes, mood swings, and weight gain. Exercise has been shown to improve mood, reduce stress, and promote better sleep quality. It also helps maintain bone density and muscle mass, which can be beneficial in preventing osteoporosis and maintaining overall strength and mobility.

A balanced diet is equally important during menopause. Women should focus on consuming nutrient-dense foods that provide essential vitamins and minerals. Calcium and vitamin D are particularly important for bone health, so women should ensure they are getting an adequate amount of these nutrients. Additionally, consuming a variety of fruits, vegetables, whole grains, lean proteins, and healthy fats can support overall health and well-being.

Stress management techniques are essential during menopause as hormonal fluctuations can contribute to increased stress levels. Practices such as meditation, deep breathing exercises, yoga, and mindfulness can help reduce stress and promote relaxation. These techniques can also improve sleep quality, which is often disrupted during menopause.

Self-care practices are crucial during menopause as they allow women to prioritize their own needs and well-being. This can include activities such as taking time for oneself, engaging in hobbies or activities that bring joy, practicing self-compassion and self-acceptance, and seeking support from friends, family, or healthcare professionals. Self-care practices can help women navigate the emotional challenges of menopause and promote a sense of well-being and fulfillment.

A natural approach to menopause also emphasizes the importance of informed decision-making. Women should educate themselves about the various treatment options available for managing menopause symptoms and make decisions based on their individual needs and preferences. This may include considering hormone replacement therapy (HRT) or exploring alternative treatments such as herbal supplements or acupuncture. It is important for women to consult with healthcare professionals to ensure safety and effectiveness.

By taking a natural approach to menopause, women can avoid unnecessary medical interventions and potential side effects. While HRT can be beneficial for some women in managing severe symptoms, it is not without risks. Hormone therapy has been associated with an increased risk of certain health conditions such as breast cancer, blood clots, and heart disease. By focusing on natural approaches, women can minimize their reliance on medications and reduce potential risks.

Furthermore, a natural approach to menopause promotes empowerment and autonomy. Women have the right to make decisions about their own bodies and health. By taking an active role in

managing their menopause symptoms, women can regain a sense of control and ownership over their bodies. This can lead to increased self-confidence and a greater sense of well-being.

It is also worth noting that a natural approach to menopause is environmentally friendly. Many conventional treatments for menopause symptoms involve the use of synthetic hormones or medications that can have negative impacts on the environment. By opting for natural approaches, women can reduce their ecological footprint and contribute to a healthier planet.

In conclusion, a natural approach to menopause is of utmost importance. Menopause is a natural biological process that should be embraced and understood. By adopting a natural approach, women can honor and respect their bodies, promote overall well-being, make informed decisions, avoid unnecessary medical interventions, and regain a sense of empowerment and autonomy. Taking a natural approach also aligns with environmental sustainability. By prioritizing a healthy lifestyle, self-care practices, and informed decision-making, women can navigate the menopausal transition with greater ease and embrace this phase as a natural part of life's journey.

Chapter Two

The Menopausal Journey

Phases of Menopause

Menopause is a natural and inevitable biological process that marks the end of a woman's reproductive years. It encompasses a series of distinct phases, each characterized by specific changes in hormonal levels, physical symptoms, and emotional experiences. In this article, we will explore the various phases of menopause, shedding light on perimenopause, menopause, and postmenopause. Understanding these phases is essential for women and their healthcare providers to effectively manage the challenges and embrace the transformations that accompany this profound life transition.

•Perimenopause: The Prelude to Change

Perimenopause, often referred to as the "menopausal transition," is the preliminary phase leading up to menopause itself. It typically begins several years before menopause and is characterized by hormonal fluctuations and a range of symptoms:

1. Irregular Periods: During perimenopause, menstrual cycles become erratic. Periods may be shorter, longer, heavier, or lighter than usual.
2. Hormonal Fluctuations: Estrogen and progesterone levels start to decline, causing irregular hormone patterns that lead to symptoms such as hot flashes, mood swings, and sleep disturbances.
3. Physical Symptoms: Women may experience changes in libido, vaginal dryness, breast tenderness, and fatigue.
4. **Emotional Changes:** Mood swings, irritability, and feelings of anxiety or depression are common due to hormonal shifts.

•Menopause: The Milestone

Menopause is officially declared when a woman has not had a menstrual period for 12 consecutive months. It is a natural biological event that marks the end of reproductive capacity. Key features of menopause include:

1. Cessation of Menstruation: The hallmark of menopause is the cessation of menstrual periods, indicating that the ovaries have stopped releasing eggs and producing significant amounts of estrogen and progesterone.

2. Hormonal Shifts: With the ovaries producing fewer hormones, menopausal symptoms such as hot flashes, night sweats, and vaginal dryness can intensify.
3. Bone Health Concerns: Reduced estrogen levels put women at a higher risk of developing osteoporosis, a condition characterized by weakened bones.
4. Cardiovascular Health: The decrease in estrogen also affects cardiovascular health, potentially increasing the risk of heart disease.

•Postmenopause: A New Phase

Postmenopause begins after menopause and continues throughout the rest of a woman's life. It is a phase characterized by steadier hormone levels and a focus on maintaining overall health:

1. Stabilization of Symptoms: Many menopausal symptoms, such as hot flashes, may diminish in severity during postmenopause.
2. Health Considerations: Postmenopausal women are at an increased risk of osteoporosis and heart disease due to decreased estrogen levels. Regular exercise, a balanced diet, and bone-strengthening activities are crucial during this phase.
3. Gynecological Health: Regular gynecological check-ups remain important to monitor any changes in vaginal health or other reproductive concerns.
4. Long-Term Health: Women should focus on preventive measures, such as maintaining a healthy weight, managing stress, and staying physically active to minimize the risk of chronic conditions associated with aging.

•The Emotional Landscape: Navigating Psychological Changes

Throughout all phases of menopause, emotional well-being plays a significant role. The hormonal fluctuations can impact mood, cognition, and overall mental health:

1. Mood Swings and Irritability: Hormonal shifts can contribute to mood swings and irritability, affecting interpersonal relationships.

2. Anxiety and Depression: Some women experience increased levels of anxiety and depression during perimenopause and menopause due to hormonal changes and the psychological impact of transitioning.
3. Cognitive Changes: "Brain fog" and memory lapses are common during menopause, often attributed to hormonal fluctuations.

•Navigating the Journey: Strategies for Each Phase

1. Perimenopause: Embracing self-care practices, such as regular exercise, a balanced diet, stress reduction techniques, and adequate sleep, can alleviate perimenopausal symptoms.

2. Menopause: Women can explore natural approaches, hormone replacement therapy (HRT), and other medical interventions to manage menopausal symptoms effectively. Consulting healthcare providers to determine the best approach is essential.
3. Postmenopause: Prioritizing heart health, bone health, and overall well-being through lifestyle modifications and regular medical check-ups is crucial for maintaining quality of life.

The journey through menopause encompasses distinct phases, each with its own challenges, experiences, and opportunities for growth. Understanding perimenopause, menopause, and postmenopause empowers women to navigate this transition with greater resilience and awareness. By seeking knowledge, adopting healthy habits, and collaborating with healthcare providers, women can embrace the transformative journey of menopause and enter the next chapter of their lives with confidence and vitality.

Common Symptoms and Challenges

Menopause, a natural and inevitable phase in a woman's life, ushers in a series of physiological, psychological, and emotional changes. While every woman's experience of menopause is unique, there are common symptoms and challenges that many encounter during this transition. In this article, we delve into the array of symptoms and complexities that women may face as they navigate the intricate landscape of menopause. By understanding these challenges, individuals and their healthcare providers can better manage and alleviate the impact of menopausal symptoms on overall well-being.

•Physical Symptoms: The Body's Expression of Change

1. Hot Flashes and Night Sweats: Among the most recognizable symptoms, hot flashes manifest as sudden waves of heat, often accompanied by sweating and a flushed complexion. These can disrupt sleep and daily activities. Night sweats, occurring during sleep, can lead to disrupted rest.
2. Irregular Periods: Perimenopause often brings erratic menstrual cycles, with periods becoming irregular in frequency, flow, and duration. Eventually, periods cease altogether as menopause is reached.
3. Vaginal Changes: The reduction of estrogen levels can lead to vaginal dryness, thinning of vaginal walls, and discomfort during intercourse. These changes may contribute to decreased libido and affect sexual satisfaction.
4. Urinary Symptoms: Some women experience increased urinary urgency, frequency, or incontinence during menopause, potentially attributed to changes in pelvic floor muscles and tissues.
5. Sleep Disturbances: Hormonal fluctuations and night sweats can disrupt sleep patterns, leading to insomnia and daytime fatigue.
6. Weight Gain and Metabolic Changes: Hormonal changes can affect metabolism, leading to shifts in body composition and weight gain, often around the abdomen.

•Emotional and Psychological Challenges

1. Mood Swings and Irritability: Fluctuating hormone levels can trigger mood swings, irritability, and emotional sensitivity. These emotional shifts can strain relationships and impact daily interactions.
2. Anxiety and Depression: Some women experience increased levels of anxiety and depression during menopause due to hormonal changes and the psychological impact of transitioning.
3. Cognitive Changes: Often termed "brain fog," cognitive changes can include memory lapses, difficulties with concentration, and a sense of mental fogginess.

•Physical and Emotional Fatigue

Physical and emotional fatigue are common symptoms experienced by many women during menopause. These symptoms can be attributed to the hormonal changes that occur during this phase.

Physical fatigue refers to a general feeling of tiredness, lack of energy, and decreased stamina. It can make simple tasks feel more challenging and can impact a woman's overall quality of life. Some women may also experience muscle aches and joint pain, which can contribute to physical fatigue.

Emotional fatigue, on the other hand, refers to feelings of mental exhaustion, irritability, mood swings, and difficulty concentrating. Hormonal fluctuations during menopause can affect neurotransmitters in the brain, leading to these emotional symptoms. Additionally, sleep disturbances, such as insomnia or night sweats, can further contribute to emotional fatigue.

Both physical and emotional fatigue can have a significant impact on a woman's daily life and well-being. They can affect her ability to perform daily activities, maintain relationships, and engage in hobbies or interests. Fatigue during menopause can also lead to increased stress levels and feelings of frustration or sadness.

Managing physical and emotional fatigue during menopause often involves a combination of lifestyle changes and medical interventions. Here are some strategies that may help:

1. Prioritize sleep: Establish a regular sleep routine and create a conducive sleep environment. Avoid caffeine and electronic devices before bedtime.
2. Exercise regularly: Engaging in regular physical activity can help boost energy levels, improve mood, and reduce fatigue. Choose activities that you enjoy and that fit your fitness level.
3. Eat a balanced diet: A nutritious diet rich in fruits, vegetables, whole grains, lean proteins, and healthy fats can provide the necessary nutrients to support energy levels.
4. Manage stress: Practice stress-reducing techniques such as deep breathing exercises, meditation, yoga, or engaging in activities that bring you joy and relaxation.
5. Seek support: Share your experiences with trusted friends or family members who can provide emotional support. Consider joining support groups or seeking professional counseling if needed.
6. Hormone replacement therapy (HRT): In some cases, healthcare providers may recommend HRT to alleviate menopausal symptoms, including fatigue. HRT involves the use of medications that replace the hormones no longer produced by the ovaries.

It is important to consult with a healthcare provider to determine the most appropriate treatment options for managing physical and emotional fatigue during menopause. They can provide personalized advice based on your specific symptoms, medical history, and individual needs.

•Challenges with Body Image and Identity

1. Body Image Concerns: Changes in body composition and weight distribution can lead to body image concerns, impacting self-esteem and self-confidence.
2. Identity Shifts: Menopause can trigger feelings of loss and identity shifts, as women grapple with the transition from reproductive years to a new phase of life.

•Social and Relationship Dynamics

1. Intimate Relationships: Vaginal dryness and decreased libido can affect intimate relationships. Open communication and exploring alternative ways of connecting can be important.
2. Social Dynamics: Mood swings and irritability can impact social interactions, potentially leading to misunderstandings with friends and family.

•Coping with Work and Daily Responsibilities

1. Workplace Challenges: Menopausal symptoms can impact work performance and concentration. Fatigue, mood swings, and cognitive changes might affect professional interactions and decision-making.
2. Daily Life Balance: Juggling menopausal symptoms with family responsibilities, career demands, and personal well-being can be challenging.

•Osteoporosis and Cardiovascular Health Concerns

Osteoporosis and cardiovascular health concerns are two common health issues that can arise during menopause.

Osteoporosis is a condition characterized by a decrease in bone density, making bones more fragile and susceptible to fractures. During menopause, the decline in estrogen levels can accelerate bone loss, leading to an increased risk of osteoporosis. Women may experience symptoms such as back pain, loss of height, and fractures, particularly in the hips, wrists, and spine.

To maintain bone health during menopause, it is important to engage in weight-bearing exercises, such as walking or strength training, which help strengthen bones. Additionally, ensuring an adequate intake of calcium and vitamin D through diet or supplements can support bone health. In some cases, healthcare providers may recommend medications called bisphosphonates or hormone therapy to prevent or treat osteoporosis.

Cardiovascular health concerns also become more prevalent during menopause. Estrogen has a protective effect on the cardiovascular system, and its decline during menopause can increase the risk of heart disease. Women may experience symptoms such as high blood pressure, high cholesterol levels, and an increased risk of developing blood clots.

To maintain cardiovascular health during menopause, it is important to adopt heart-healthy lifestyle habits. This includes eating a balanced diet low in saturated fats and cholesterol, engaging in regular physical activity, maintaining a healthy weight, avoiding smoking, and managing stress levels. Regular check-ups with a healthcare provider are also important to monitor blood pressure, cholesterol levels, and other cardiovascular risk factors. In some cases, healthcare providers may recommend medications such as statins or hormone therapy to manage cardiovascular health concerns during menopause.

Overall, menopause is a time of significant hormonal changes that can impact various aspects of a woman's health. It is important to prioritize self-care, seek medical advice when needed, and make lifestyle changes to support physical and emotional well-being during this transitional phase.

•Seeking Solutions: Coping Strategies and Support

1. Lifestyle Modifications: Regular exercise, a balanced diet, stress management techniques, and adequate sleep can help alleviate a range of menopausal symptoms.
2. Hormone Replacement Therapy (HRT): Some women opt for HRT to manage severe symptoms. It involves replacing hormones no longer produced in sufficient amounts.
3. Natural Remedies: Herbal supplements, acupuncture, and mindfulness practices are explored by some as alternatives to manage symptoms.
4. Communication and Support: Engaging in open conversations with healthcare providers, partners, friends, and family can provide emotional support and practical solutions.

Menopause is a multifaceted journey characterized by a diverse array of symptoms and challenges. By understanding these complexities, women and their healthcare providers can collaboratively develop strategies to manage and alleviate the impact of menopausal symptoms. Embracing lifestyle modifications, seeking professional guidance, nurturing emotional well-being, and fostering a supportive environment are key steps in navigating the challenges of menopause. By doing so, women can transition through this transformative phase with resilience, empowerment, and a renewed sense of well-being.

Chapter Three

Nurturing Your Body

Nutrition for Menopause

As women navigate the intricate terrain of menopause, the importance of a balanced and supportive diet cannot be overstated. Menopause brings about hormonal shifts and physiological changes that can impact overall well-being. Proper nutrition during this phase plays a vital role in managing symptoms, maintaining bone health, supporting cardiovascular function, and promoting emotional equilibrium. In this article, we delve into the significance of nutrition for menopause and explore dietary strategies to empower women to thrive during this transformative life stage.

•Understanding Menopause and its Impact on Nutrition

Menopause is characterized by the natural cessation of menstruation and a decline in reproductive hormones, particularly estrogen. This hormonal shift influences various aspects of a woman's body, including metabolism, bone health, cardiovascular function, and emotional well-being. Proper nutrition can mitigate the effects of these changes and optimize health outcomes.

•Bone Health: Calcium and Vitamin D

Bone health is a significant concern during menopause due to the decline in estrogen levels, which can lead to a loss of bone density and an increased risk of osteoporosis. Calcium and vitamin D play crucial roles in maintaining bone health and should be prioritized in the diet during menopause.

Calcium is a mineral that is essential for building and maintaining strong bones. It is important to consume an adequate amount of calcium to support bone health, as well as other functions in the body. Good food sources of calcium include dairy products such as milk, yogurt, and cheese, as well as leafy green vegetables like kale and broccoli. Additionally, fortified plant-based milk alternatives such as almond milk or soy milk can also provide calcium.

Vitamin D is necessary for the absorption of calcium in the body. It helps regulate calcium levels and promotes bone mineralization. The primary source of vitamin D is sunlight exposure, as the skin produces vitamin D when exposed to sunlight. However, during menopause, it may be challenging to obtain sufficient vitamin D from sunlight alone. Therefore, it is recommended to include dietary sources of vitamin D in the diet. Fatty fish like salmon and mackerel are excellent sources of vitamin D. Additionally, fortified foods such as milk, orange juice, and breakfast cereals can provide vitamin D as well.

It is important to note that calcium and vitamin D work together synergistically to support bone health. Adequate intake of both nutrients is necessary for optimal bone health during menopause. The recommended daily intake of calcium for women over 50 years old is 1200 mg, while the recommended daily intake of vitamin D is 600-800 IU.

In some cases, it may be challenging to meet the recommended intake of calcium and vitamin D through diet alone. In these instances, supplements may be beneficial. Calcium supplements are available in various forms, such as calcium carbonate or calcium citrate. It is important to choose a supplement that is easily absorbed by the body. Vitamin D supplements are also available and can be taken if sunlight exposure or dietary sources are insufficient.

However, it is essential to consult with a healthcare provider or registered dietitian before starting any new supplements, as individual needs may vary. They can assess your specific needs and recommend the appropriate dosage and form of supplements for you.

In conclusion, calcium and vitamin D are crucial for maintaining bone health during menopause. Adequate intake of calcium-rich foods and dietary sources of vitamin D, along with sunlight exposure, is recommended. Supplements may be necessary in some cases, but it is important to seek professional guidance before starting any new supplements.

•Heart Health: Omega-3 Fatty Acids and Fiber

Heart health is also an important consideration during menopause. Omega-3 fatty acids and fiber can play a significant role in supporting heart health during this time.

Omega-3 fatty acids are a type of polyunsaturated fat that has been shown to have numerous cardiovascular benefits. They can help reduce inflammation, lower triglyceride levels, decrease blood pressure, and improve overall heart health. Good food sources of omega-3 fatty acids include fatty fish like salmon, sardines, and mackerel, as well as walnuts, flaxseeds, and chia seeds. Including these foods in the diet can help support heart health during menopause.

Fiber is another important nutrient for heart health. It can help lower cholesterol levels, regulate blood sugar levels, and promote healthy digestion. High-fiber foods include whole grains like oats, quinoa, and brown rice, as well as fruits, vegetables, legumes, and nuts. Including a variety of these fiber-rich foods in the diet can help support heart health and overall well-being during menopause.

In addition to consuming omega-3 fatty acids and fiber, it is also important to maintain a healthy lifestyle during menopause. This includes regular physical activity, managing stress levels, getting enough sleep, and avoiding smoking and excessive alcohol consumption. These lifestyle factors, combined with a balanced diet rich in omega-3 fatty acids and fiber, can contribute to optimal heart health during menopause.

It is worth noting that individual needs may vary, and it is always beneficial to consult with a healthcare provider or registered dietitian for personalized advice on maintaining heart health during menopause. They can assess your specific needs and provide recommendations tailored to your unique situation.

•Weight Management and Metabolism

Weight management and metabolism can be challenging during menopause due to hormonal changes and age-related factors. Many women experience weight gain, particularly in the abdominal area, during this time. This can be attributed to a decrease in estrogen levels, which can lead to a redistribution of fat from the hips and thighs to the abdomen.

Slowing metabolism is another common issue during menopause. As women age, their metabolism naturally slows down, making it easier to gain weight and harder to lose it. This can be frustrating for women who may have previously been able to maintain their weight with less effort.

However, there are strategies that can help manage weight and support a healthy metabolism during menopause:

1. Balanced diet: Eating a balanced diet that includes lean proteins, whole grains, fruits, vegetables, and healthy fats is important for maintaining a healthy weight and supporting metabolism. It is also important to be mindful of portion sizes and avoid excessive calorie intake.
2. Regular physical activity: Engaging in regular physical activity is crucial for managing weight and boosting metabolism. Incorporating a combination of aerobic exercise, strength training, and flexibility exercises can help maintain muscle mass, which can help support a healthy metabolism.
3. Strength training: Including strength training exercises in your fitness routine can be particularly beneficial during menopause. Building muscle mass through strength training can help increase metabolism and burn more calories even at rest.
4. Managing stress: Chronic stress can contribute to weight gain and hinder weight loss efforts. Finding healthy ways to manage stress, such as through exercise, relaxation techniques, or engaging in enjoyable activities, can be helpful for maintaining a healthy weight during menopause.
5. Adequate sleep: Getting enough quality sleep is important for weight management and metabolism. Lack of sleep can disrupt hormone levels and increase appetite, leading to weight gain. Aim for seven to nine hours of sleep per night.
6. Hormone therapy: In some cases, hormone therapy may be recommended to manage menopausal symptoms. It is important to discuss the potential benefits and risks of hormone therapy with a healthcare provider.

It is important to remember that weight management and metabolism can be complex and individualized during menopause. Consulting with a healthcare provider or registered dietitian

can provide personalized guidance and support for managing weight and supporting a healthy metabolism during this time.

•Hormone-Balancing Foods and Phytoestrogens

1. Phytoestrogens: Found in soy products, flaxseeds, chickpeas, and lentils, phytoestrogens are plant compounds that can mimic estrogen's effects in the body. They may help alleviate some menopausal symptoms.
2. Soy Products: Consuming moderate amounts of whole soy foods, such as tofu and tempeh, has been associated with potential benefits for hot flashes and heart health.

•Micronutrients and Antioxidants

Micronutrients and antioxidants play an important role in overall health and can also be beneficial during menopause. Here are some key points to consider:

1. Micronutrients: During menopause, it is important to ensure adequate intake of essential vitamins and minerals. Some micronutrients that may be particularly important during this time include:

- Calcium: Menopause is associated with a higher risk of osteoporosis, so ensuring adequate calcium intake is crucial for maintaining bone health.

- Vitamin D: Vitamin D plays a role in calcium absorption and bone health. It is also involved in immune function and may have a positive impact on mood.

- Vitamin B12: Menopause can sometimes lead to decreased absorption of vitamin B12, so it is important to ensure adequate intake through food or supplements. Vitamin B12 is important for energy production and nerve function.

- Iron: Iron needs may decrease after menopause due to the cessation of menstruation. However, it is still important to monitor iron levels and ensure adequate intake, as iron deficiency can lead to fatigue and other symptoms.

2. Antioxidants: Antioxidants help protect cells from damage caused by free radicals, which are unstable molecules that can contribute to chronic diseases and aging. Some antioxidants that may be particularly beneficial during menopause include:

- Vitamin C: Vitamin C is a powerful antioxidant that supports immune function and collagen production. It can also help reduce oxidative stress.

- Vitamin E: Vitamin E is another antioxidant that can help reduce oxidative stress and support heart health. It may also have a positive impact on skin health.

- Selenium: Selenium is a mineral that acts as an antioxidant and helps support thyroid function. It can be found in foods like Brazil nuts, fish, and whole grains.

It is important to note that while a balanced diet should provide most of the necessary micronutrients and antioxidants, some women may benefit from supplementation. Consulting with a healthcare provider or registered dietitian can help determine individual needs and provide personalized recommendations.

Overall, focusing on a varied and nutrient-dense diet that includes a wide range of fruits, vegetables, whole grains, lean proteins, and healthy fats can help ensure adequate intake of micronutrients and antioxidants during menopause.

•Hydration and Herbal Teas

Hydration is important for overall health, and it becomes even more crucial during menopause. As women age, their bodies may become less efficient at regulating fluid balance, leading to an increased risk of dehydration. Additionally, menopausal symptoms such as hot flashes and night sweats can contribute to fluid loss.

Drinking an adequate amount of water throughout the day is essential for maintaining hydration. The general recommendation is to aim for about 8 cups (64 ounces) of water per day, but individual needs may vary depending on factors such as activity level and climate.

In addition to water, herbal teas can be a hydrating and beneficial option during menopause. Some herbal teas may also offer additional health benefits:

- Peppermint tea: Peppermint tea can help soothe digestive issues, such as bloating and indigestion, which can be common during menopause.

- Chamomile tea: Chamomile tea has calming properties and may help promote relaxation and better sleep, which can be beneficial for managing menopausal symptoms like anxiety and insomnia.

- Red clover tea: Red clover tea contains isoflavones, which are plant compounds that have estrogen-like effects in the body. These compounds may help alleviate menopausal symptoms such as hot flashes and night sweats.

- Sage tea: Sage tea has been traditionally used to reduce excessive sweating and hot flashes. It may also have antimicrobial properties.

It is important to note that some herbal teas may interact with certain medications or have potential side effects. It is always a good idea to consult with a healthcare provider before incorporating herbal teas into your routine, especially if you have any underlying health conditions or take medications.

Overall, staying hydrated and incorporating herbal teas into your daily routine can be beneficial during menopause. However, it is important to prioritize water intake and choose herbal teas wisely based on your individual needs and preferences.

•Embracing a Balanced Approach: Key Takeaways

1. Variety: Incorporate a wide variety of foods to ensure a well-rounded nutrient intake.
2. Moderation: Enjoy foods in moderation, especially those high in added sugars and unhealthy fats.

3. Whole Foods: Prioritize whole, minimally processed foods over heavily processed options.
4. Mindful Eating: Pay attention to hunger and fullness cues, and eat mindfully to support digestion.
5. Consult a Healthcare Provider: If considering supplements, consult a healthcare provider to determine individual needs and avoid excessive intakes.

•Personalized Nutrition for Menopause

Personalized nutrition for menopause involves tailoring dietary choices to meet the specific needs and challenges that women may face during this stage of life. Here are some key considerations for personalized nutrition during menopause:

1. Calcium and vitamin D: Menopause is associated with a decline in estrogen levels, which can lead to a decrease in bone density and an increased risk of osteoporosis. Adequate calcium and vitamin D intake is essential for maintaining bone health. Good sources of calcium include dairy products, leafy green vegetables, and fortified foods. Vitamin D can be obtained through sun exposure or from dietary sources such as fatty fish and fortified foods.
2. Phytoestrogens: Phytoestrogens are plant compounds that have estrogen-like effects in the body. They may help alleviate menopausal symptoms such as hot flashes and night sweats. Foods rich in phytoestrogens include soy products, flaxseeds, and legumes.
3. Omega-3 fatty acids: Omega-3 fatty acids have anti-inflammatory properties and may help reduce the risk of heart disease, which becomes more prevalent after menopause. Good sources of omega-3 fatty acids include fatty fish, flaxseeds, chia seeds, and walnuts.
4. Fiber: Menopause is associated with changes in metabolism and weight gain. Consuming an adequate amount of fiber can help promote satiety, regulate blood sugar levels, and support digestive health. Good sources of fiber include whole grains, fruits, vegetables, legumes, and nuts.
5. Limiting processed foods and added sugars: Menopause is a time when women may be more prone to weight gain and metabolic changes. It is important to limit the

   consumption of processed foods and added sugars, as they can contribute to weight gain, inflammation, and an increased risk of chronic diseases.
6. Hydration: As mentioned earlier, staying hydrated is crucial during menopause. Drinking an adequate amount of water and incorporating hydrating herbal teas can help maintain fluid balance and alleviate symptoms such as hot flashes and night sweats.

It is important to note that personalized nutrition during menopause should take into account individual preferences, dietary restrictions, and any underlying health conditions. Consulting with a registered dietitian or healthcare provider can help create a personalized nutrition plan that meets specific needs and goals during this stage of life.

A nourishing diet is a cornerstone of well-being during menopause, supporting bone health, heart health, weight management, and overall vitality. By embracing a balanced and nutrient-rich approach to nutrition, women can harness the power of food to navigate the challenges of menopause with resilience, optimize their health, and embark on a journey of positive transformation.

Hormone-Balancing Foods

The transition through menopause is a transformative journey marked by hormonal shifts that can bring about a variety of physical and emotional changes. Hormone imbalances during this phase can lead to symptoms such as hot flashes, mood swings, and disrupted sleep. While medical interventions exist, exploring a natural approach through hormone-balancing foods can offer a complementary strategy for managing these changes. In this article, we delve into the world of hormone-balancing foods and their potential to promote well-being during menopause.

•The Hormonal Landscape of Menopause

Menopause involves a decline in the production of estrogen and progesterone, the two key reproductive hormones. This shift can lead to hormonal imbalances that contribute to a range of symptoms, including:

1. Hot Flashes: Sudden feelings of warmth and intense sweating.

2. Mood Swings: Emotional fluctuations, irritability, and anxiety.

3. Sleep Disturbances: Insomnia and disrupted sleep patterns.

4. Vaginal Dryness: Reduced vaginal lubrication and discomfort during intercourse.

5. Bone Health Concerns: Decreased estrogen levels can impact bone density.

6. Metabolic Changes: Hormonal changes can affect metabolism and weight management.

•Harnessing Hormone-Balancing Foods

Certain foods contain compounds that can influence hormone balance, alleviate symptoms, and promote overall well-being during menopause. Incorporating these foods into your diet can have a positive impact on your hormonal health.

-Phytoestrogens: Plant Compounds with Hormonal Effects

Phytoestrogens are naturally occurring plant compounds that can mimic the effects of estrogen in the body. By binding to estrogen receptors, they can help regulate hormonal imbalances. Examples of phytoestrogen-rich foods include:

1. Soy Products: Tofu, tempeh, soy milk, and edamame are rich sources of phytoestrogens called isoflavones. They may help alleviate hot flashes and support bone health.
2. Flaxseeds: Flaxseeds are high in lignans, a type of phytoestrogen. Ground flaxseeds can be added to yogurt, smoothies, or baked goods for a hormone-balancing boost.
3. Legumes: Beans, lentils, and chickpeas are not only rich in fiber but also contain phytoestrogens that support hormonal balance.

-Cruciferous Vegetables: Detoxification and Balance

Cruciferous vegetables contain compounds called indoles that aid in hormone metabolism and detoxification. These vegetables include:

1. Broccoli: Rich in indole-3-carbinol, which supports estrogen metabolism and may reduce the risk of certain cancers.
2. Cauliflower: Contains indoles that help maintain hormonal balance.
3. Cabbage: Offers similar benefits, supporting healthy estrogen levels.

-Omega-3 Fatty Acids: Anti-Inflammatory Support

Omega-3 fatty acids possess anti-inflammatory properties that can help manage inflammation-related symptoms. Foods rich in omega-3s include:

1. Fatty Fish: Salmon, mackerel, sardines, and trout are excellent sources of omega-3s.
2. Flaxseeds and Walnuts: These plant-based sources provide alpha-linolenic acid (ALA), a type of omega-3.

-Antioxidant-Rich Foods: Cellular Protection

Antioxidants help protect cells from oxidative stress and inflammation. Incorporate antioxidant-rich foods into your diet:

1. Berries: Blueberries, strawberries, and raspberries are rich in antioxidants.

2. Colorful Vegetables: Bell peppers, sweet potatoes, and carrots provide a spectrum of antioxidants.

-Healthy Fats: Balance and Hormone Production

Healthy fats play a role in hormone production and overall well-being. Sources of healthy fats include:

1. Avocado: Rich in monounsaturated fats that support hormone production.
2. Nuts and Seeds: Almonds, walnuts, and chia seeds provide healthy fats and other nutrients.

-Whole Grains: Steady Energy and Fiber

Whole grains offer sustained energy and fiber that supports blood sugar balance and digestive health:

1. Quinoa: Contains protein, fiber, and essential nutrients.
2. Oats: Rich in soluble fiber, which can aid in cholesterol management.

-Flavorful Herbs and Spices: Natural Support

Certain herbs and spices can contribute to hormonal balance and overall well-being:

1. Turmeric: Contains curcumin, known for its anti-inflammatory properties.
2. Cinnamon: May help regulate blood sugar levels and support metabolic health.

•Incorporating Hormone-Balancing Foods into Your Diet

1. Balance and Variety: Aim for a well-rounded diet that includes a variety of hormone-balancing foods.
2. Daily Intake: Incorporate a serving of phytoestrogen-rich foods, cruciferous vegetables, omega-3 sources, and antioxidant-rich foods daily.

3. Mindful Preparation: Experiment with recipes that showcase hormone-balancing ingredients in delicious and satisfying ways.

•Consultation and Personalization

Consultation and personalization are important aspects of hormonal therapy in menopause. During a consultation, a healthcare provider will assess an individual's specific needs and symptoms to determine the most appropriate hormonal therapy options. Personalization involves tailoring the treatment plan to address the unique needs and preferences of each individual. This may include adjusting the dosage, type of hormone therapy, or delivery method to optimize effectiveness and minimize side effects. It's crucial to consult with a healthcare professional for personalized advice on hormonal therapy in menopause.

As women navigate the dynamic landscape of menopause, harnessing the power of hormone-balancing foods can contribute to a smoother journey. Phytoestrogens, cruciferous vegetables, omega-3s, antioxidants, and other nutrient-dense options offer natural support for hormonal balance, symptom management, and overall well-being. By incorporating these foods into a well-rounded diet, women can embrace the transformative experience of menopause with vitality and resilience.

Herbal Support and Supplements

As individuals seek holistic approaches to manage the challenges of menopause, herbal support and supplements have gained prominence for their potential to alleviate symptoms and promote well-being. In this article, we delve into the world of herbal remedies and supplements for menopause, exploring their benefits, potential risks, and considerations for incorporating them into a holistic approach to health during this transformative journey.

•The Appeal of Herbal Support and Supplements

Herbs and supplements offer a natural and holistic approach to managing menopause-related symptoms. Many women are drawn to these alternatives due to concerns about conventional treatments, such as hormone replacement therapy (HRT), and a desire for more personalized and gentle solutions.

•Popular Herbal Remedies for Menopause

1. Black Cohosh: Widely studied for its potential to reduce hot flashes and night sweats, black cohosh is believed to have estrogen-like effects.
2. Red Clover: Containing compounds called isoflavones, red clover may offer relief from hot flashes and other menopausal symptoms.
3. Sage: This herb has a reputation for reducing night sweats and promoting emotional well-being.
4. Dong Quai: A traditional Chinese herb, dong quai is believed to help balance hormones and alleviate menopausal symptoms.
5. Ginseng: Known for its adaptogenic properties, ginseng may help manage stress and improve energy levels.
6. Chasteberry (Vitex): Chasteberry may support hormonal balance by influencing the pituitary gland, which regulates hormone production.

•Understanding Herbal Supplements

Understanding herbal supplements in menopause involves recognizing the appeal they hold for women seeking natural remedies and alternative options to manage menopausal symptoms. Many women turn to herbal supplements as a way to alleviate symptoms such as hot flashes, night sweats, mood swings, and sleep disturbances without relying on hormone replacement therapy (HRT) or prescription medications.

The appeal of herbal supplements lies in their natural origins and the belief that they may provide relief without the potential risks and side effects associated with pharmaceutical interventions. Women often prefer to explore herbal options as a more holistic and gentler approach to managing their menopausal symptoms.

Some popular herbal supplements used during menopause include black cohosh, red clover, dong quai, maca root, and evening primrose oil. These herbs are believed to have estrogen-like effects or help regulate hormonal imbalances, which can contribute to the alleviation of symptoms such as hot flashes, night sweats, vaginal dryness, mood swings, and low libido.

Black cohosh is commonly used to relieve hot flashes and night sweats, while red clover contains isoflavones that are similar to estrogen and may help reduce hot flashes and improve bone

density. Dong quai, a herb used in traditional Chinese medicine, is believed to have estrogen-like effects and may alleviate hot flashes, vaginal dryness, and mood swings. Maca root is often used to balance hormones and improve energy levels, potentially reducing hot flashes, improving mood, and enhancing libido. Evening primrose oil contains gamma-linolenic acid (GLA), which may help relieve breast pain and tenderness associated with menopause.

However, it is important to approach herbal supplements with caution. The effectiveness and safety of these supplements are not well-regulated or supported by extensive scientific research. There is limited evidence regarding their efficacy and potential side effects. Additionally, herbal supplements can interact with medications or have their own side effects. Therefore, it is crucial to consult with a healthcare provider before starting any new supplement regimen.

Furthermore, it is essential to recognize that herbal supplements may not work for everyone. Menopause is a highly individual experience, and what works for one person may not work for another. It is important for women to explore different options and find what works best for their unique needs and preferences. This may involve a combination of herbal supplements, lifestyle changes, and other interventions tailored to their specific symptoms and overall health.

•Potential Benefits of Herbal Support and Supplements

1. Alleviating Menopausal Symptoms: Certain herbs, such as black cohosh and red clover, have shown promise in reducing hot flashes, night sweats, and mood disturbances.
2. Natural Hormone Balancing: Some herbs, like chasteberry and dong quai, are believed to help regulate hormonal fluctuations.
3. Emotional Support: Herbs like sage and ginseng may promote emotional well-being and stress management.
4. Bone Health: Certain supplements, such as calcium and vitamin D, can help support bone density during and after menopause.

•Considerations and Potential Risks

1. Individual Responses: Responses to herbs and supplements can vary widely, and what works for one person may not work for another.
2. Interactions: Some herbs and supplements may interact with medications or other supplements, leading to potential adverse effects.
3. Dosage and Duration: It's crucial to follow recommended dosages and not exceed them. Long-term use of certain supplements may have unknown effects.
4. Quality Control: The quality and potency of herbal supplements can vary. Choose products from reputable sources and manufacturers.

•Holistic Approach: Integrating Herbal Support

1. Consultation: Always consult a healthcare provider before introducing new herbs or supplements into your routine, especially if you have underlying health conditions or are taking medications.

2. Holistic Consideration: Herbal remedies should complement, not replace, a holistic approach that includes proper nutrition, exercise, stress management, and emotional support.
3. Trial Period: When trying a new herbal remedy or supplement, consider keeping a journal to track its effects and any changes in symptoms.
4. Patience: Natural remedies may take time to show results. Be patient and allow sufficient time for the herbs or supplements to have an effect.

As women navigate the intricate terrain of menopause, herbal support and supplements offer a natural pathway to managing symptoms and promoting overall well-being. While herbal remedies hold promise, it's crucial to approach them with informed awareness, understanding potential benefits and risks, and seeking guidance from healthcare providers. By integrating herbal support within a comprehensive and holistic approach to menopause management, women can embark on this transformative journey with confidence, empowerment, and a sense of balance.

Chapter Four

Mind-Body Wellness

Managing Stress and Emotional Changes

Menopause, a significant life transition, brings about not only physical changes but also a range of emotional shifts that can impact a woman's overall well-being. The hormonal fluctuations accompanying menopause can contribute to mood swings, irritability, anxiety, and other emotional challenges. Managing stress and emotional changes is crucial for navigating this transformative journey with resilience and balance. In this article, we delve into the emotional landscape of menopause and explore effective strategies for managing stress and promoting emotional well-being during this phase of life.

•The Emotional Landscape of Menopause

The emotional landscape of menopause is complex and can vary greatly from woman to woman. Menopause is a significant life transition that marks the end of a woman's reproductive years, and it can bring about a range of emotions and psychological changes.

One of the most commonly reported emotional symptoms of menopause is mood swings. Hormonal fluctuations during this time can lead to irritability, anxiety, and feelings of sadness or depression. These mood swings can be unpredictable and may occur without any apparent trigger. They can impact a woman's overall well-being and relationships, causing stress and strain on both personal and professional levels.

Another emotional aspect of menopause is the potential for increased feelings of self-doubt and decreased self-esteem. As women experience physical changes such as weight gain, changes in body shape, and skin changes, they may feel less confident in their appearance and struggle with body image issues. This can contribute to feelings of insecurity and a loss of self-worth.

Menopause can also bring about a sense of loss or grief. The end of fertility and the realization that one's childbearing years are over can be emotionally challenging for some women. This loss of a significant phase of life can lead to feelings of sadness, nostalgia, or even a sense of identity crisis.

Additionally, menopause can have an impact on sexuality and intimacy. Hormonal changes during this time can lead to vaginal dryness, decreased libido, and discomfort during sexual activity. These physical changes, coupled with the emotional challenges of menopause, can affect a woman's sexual confidence and desire, potentially straining intimate relationships.

It is important to note that not all women will experience these emotional symptoms to the same degree or at all. Some women may navigate menopause with relative ease, while others may find

it more emotionally challenging. Each woman's experience is unique, and it is important to validate and support individual experiences.

Managing the emotional landscape of menopause often involves a multifaceted approach. This may include seeking support from healthcare providers, therapists, or support groups to address emotional concerns and develop coping strategies. Engaging in self-care practices such as exercise, relaxation techniques, and maintaining a healthy lifestyle can also help manage emotional symptoms. Additionally, open communication with partners and loved ones can foster understanding and support during this time of transition.

Overall, recognizing and addressing the emotional aspects of menopause is crucial for women to navigate this phase of life with resilience and well-being. By acknowledging and seeking support for emotional changes, women can enhance their overall quality of life during menopause.

•Stress and Menopause: A Complex Relationship

Stress and menopause have a complex relationship that can impact a woman's emotional well-being during this transitional phase. Menopause itself can be a stressful experience due to the physical and hormonal changes that occur. Additionally, the emotional symptoms of menopause, such as mood swings and feelings of self-doubt, can further contribute to stress levels.

Stress can also have a reciprocal relationship with menopause, meaning that menopause itself can be a stressor that exacerbates existing stress levels. The hormonal fluctuations during menopause can affect the body's stress response system, leading to increased feelings of stress and anxiety. This can create a cycle where stress worsens menopausal symptoms, and menopausal symptoms contribute to increased stress levels.

The physiological changes that occur during menopause can also make women more vulnerable to stress. For example, hot flashes and night sweats can disrupt sleep patterns, leading to fatigue and increased irritability. Sleep disturbances and fatigue can make it more difficult for women to cope with daily stressors, leading to a heightened sense of stress and overwhelm.

Additionally, the emotional challenges of menopause, such as feelings of sadness or loss, can be stressful in themselves. Women may experience stress related to the changes in their identity and the uncertainty of navigating this new phase of life. The impact on sexuality and intimacy can also create stress within relationships.

Managing stress during menopause is crucial for overall well-being. This may involve implementing stress management techniques such as relaxation exercises, mindfulness practices, or engaging in activities that promote emotional well-being, such as hobbies or spending time with loved ones. Seeking support from healthcare providers or therapists can also provide valuable tools and strategies for managing stress during this time.

It is important to note that stress management techniques may vary for each individual, and what works for one woman may not work for another. It may take some trial and error to find effective strategies for managing stress during menopause. Additionally, seeking support from loved ones and communicating openly about the challenges of menopause can help alleviate stress and foster understanding.

In conclusion, the relationship between stress and menopause is complex and can impact a woman's emotional well-being during this transitional phase. Recognizing and addressing stress during menopause is crucial for managing emotional symptoms and enhancing overall quality of life. By implementing stress management techniques and seeking support, women can navigate menopause with resilience and well-being.

•Strategies for Managing Stress and Emotional Changes

1. Mindfulness and Meditation: Cultivating Presence

Mindfulness practices, such as meditation and deep breathing exercises, help calm the mind, reduce stress, and promote emotional stability. Regular practice enhances self-awareness and enables individuals to respond to emotional changes with greater equanimity.

2. Yoga: Balancing Body and Mind
Yoga combines physical postures, breathing exercises, and meditation to promote relaxation, flexibility, and emotional balance. Practicing yoga regularly can ease tension, reduce anxiety, and enhance overall well-being.
3. Regular Exercise: Boosting Mood

Engaging in regular physical activity stimulates the release of endorphins, natural mood-enhancing chemicals. Exercise helps alleviate stress, reduce irritability, and promote emotional resilience.

4. Social Support: Nurturing Connections

Maintaining strong social connections with friends and family provides a support system during times of emotional flux. Sharing experiences and seeking empathetic conversations can alleviate feelings of isolation.

5. Healthy Diet: Nourishing the Mind

A balanced diet rich in whole foods, lean proteins, and omega-3 fatty acids supports brain health and emotional stability. Avoiding excessive caffeine, refined sugars, and processed foods can help prevent mood swings.

6. Adequate Sleep: Rejuvenating the Mind

Prioritize good sleep hygiene, such as establishing a regular sleep schedule, creating a comfortable sleep environment, and practicing relaxation techniques before bedtime.

7. Expressive Writing: Catharsis and Reflection

Journaling or expressive writing provides an outlet for processing emotions and thoughts. It can help individuals gain clarity, release pent-up feelings, and develop insights into their emotional experiences.

8. Professional Support: Seeking Guidance

If emotional changes become overwhelming or interfere with daily life, consider seeking support from mental health professionals, such as therapists or counselors.

•Mind-Body Connection: Nurturing Emotional Well-being

1. Cognitive Behavioral Therapy (CBT): Shifting Patterns

CBT is a therapeutic approach that helps individuals recognize and modify negative thought patterns. It can be particularly effective in managing anxiety and depression.

2. Biofeedback and Relaxation Techniques: Stress Management

Biofeedback involves learning to control physiological responses, such as heart rate and muscle tension. This technique can promote relaxation and stress reduction.

3. Acupuncture: Balancing Energy

Acupuncture, an ancient Chinese practice, involves inserting thin needles into specific points on the body. It is believed to balance the body's energy and promote emotional harmony.

•Self-Compassion and Resilience: A Holistic Approach

1. Self-Care Rituals: Prioritizing Personal Well-being

Engage in activities that bring joy and relaxation, whether it's taking a bath, reading a book, practicing a hobby, or spending time in nature.

2. Cultivating Resilience: Adapting to Change

Embrace change as an opportunity for growth. Developing resilience allows individuals to bounce back from emotional challenges and adapt to new circumstances.

•Hormone Replacement Therapy (HRT) and Emotional Well-being

1. Consulting a Healthcare Provider: Informed Choices

For some women, hormone replacement therapy (HRT) can help alleviate emotional changes associated with menopause. Consulting a healthcare provider to discuss the risks and benefits is essential.

2. Personalized Approach: Individual Needs

The decision to pursue HRT should be based on individual health history, preferences, and the severity of emotional symptoms.

Navigating the emotional changes and managing stress during menopause requires a holistic approach that addresses both physical and mental well-being. By integrating strategies that promote mindfulness, exercise, social support, healthy eating, and professional guidance, women can embrace the emotional shifts of menopause with resilience and grace. As each woman's journey is unique, finding a personalized combination of strategies empowers her to navigate this transformative phase with a sense of equilibrium and well-being.

Mindfulness and Meditation

Menopause, a profound life transition, brings about physical, emotional, and psychological changes that can impact a woman's overall well-being. In the midst of these shifts, the practice of mindfulness and meditation offers a valuable tool for navigating the journey with grace and resilience. Mindfulness, the art of being fully present in the moment, and meditation, a practice of cultivating inner calm and awareness, can provide profound benefits during menopause. In this article, we explore the significance of mindfulness and meditation, their potential benefits, and practical strategies for integrating these practices into the menopausal experience.

•The Menopausal Journey and Emotional Landscape

Menopause is characterized by hormonal fluctuations that can lead to a range of symptoms, including hot flashes, mood swings, and disrupted sleep. Emotional changes, such as increased

irritability, anxiety, and occasional bouts of sadness, are also common due to hormonal shifts and the significant life transition menopause represents.

•The Essence of Mindfulness and Meditation

Mindfulness involves paying non-judgmental attention to the present moment, cultivating awareness of thoughts, feelings, bodily sensations, and the surrounding environment. Meditation, on the other hand, is a focused mental practice that promotes relaxation, inner calm, and mental clarity.

•Benefits of Mindfulness and Meditation during Menopause

1. Stress Reduction: Mindfulness and meditation can help manage stress by calming the nervous system and reducing the production of stress hormones.
2. Emotional Resilience: These practices promote emotional regulation, allowing individuals to respond to emotions with greater equanimity and self-awareness.
3. Anxiety and Mood Management: Mindfulness and meditation techniques can alleviate symptoms of anxiety, depression, and mood swings.
4. Sleep Improvement: Regular practice can lead to improved sleep quality by calming the mind and reducing sleep-disrupting thoughts.
5. Cognitive Enhancement: Mindfulness has been linked to improved cognitive function, attention, and memory.
6. Physical Well-being: Meditation has been shown to lower blood pressure, improve immune function, and reduce inflammation.

•Practical Strategies for Integrating Mindfulness and Meditation

1. Breathing Awareness: Focus on your breath, observing its natural rhythm. When thoughts arise, gently bring your attention back to your breath.
2. Body Scan: Pay attention to each part of your body, noting any sensations without judgment. This practice promotes body awareness and relaxation.
3. Guided Meditations: Use audio recordings or apps that offer guided meditation sessions tailored to different purposes, such as stress reduction, sleep, or emotional balance.
4. Mindful Eating: Engage all your senses while eating, savoring each bite. Pay attention to the flavors, textures, and sensations.
5. Walking Meditation: Practice mindful walking, feeling the sensation of each step and connecting with the environment around you.
6. Journaling: Combine mindfulness with writing. Reflect on your thoughts, feelings, and experiences without judgment.

7. Mindful Pause: Take short breaks during the day to center yourself. Close your eyes, take a few deep breaths, and refocus your attention on the present moment.

•Cultivating Mindfulness in Daily Life

1. Morning Ritual: Begin your day with a few minutes of mindful breathing or meditation to set a positive tone.
2. Mindful Eating: Slow down during meals, savoring each bite and being aware of the nourishment you're providing your body.
3. Mindful Pause: When faced with stress or overwhelm, take a mindful pause to center yourself before responding.
4. Bedtime Routine: Wind down with a few minutes of relaxation, whether through gentle stretching, deep breathing, or meditation.

•Creating a Supportive Environment

1. Designating a Space: Set up a quiet and comfortable space for your mindfulness and meditation practice.
2. Time Commitment: Start with a few minutes each day and gradually increase the duration as you become more comfortable with the practice.
3. Consistency: Establish a regular routine, incorporating mindfulness and meditation into your daily schedule.
4. Gentleness and Patience: Approach your practice with kindness and patience. Embrace the journey without expecting perfection.

•Mindfulness-Based Stress Reduction (MBSR) and Menopause

1. MBSR Program: MBSR is a structured program that incorporates mindfulness meditation to reduce stress and improve well-being. Participating in an MBSR course can provide valuable tools for managing menopausal challenges.
2. Professional Guidance: Enrolling in an MBSR course led by a qualified instructor offers guidance and support for developing a sustained mindfulness practice.

Mindfulness and meditation are powerful tools that can support women through the intricate terrain of menopause. By cultivating present-moment awareness, individuals can navigate emotional changes, alleviate stress, and foster emotional resilience. Embracing these practices as an integral part of daily life offers a pathway to tranquility, self-awareness, and enhanced well-being. Through the practice of mindfulness and meditation, women can harness their inner resources to navigate menopause with grace, balance, and a sense of mindful tranquility.

Yoga and Exercise for Menopause

Menopause is a transformative phase that brings about hormonal shifts and a range of physical and emotional changes. Engaging in regular physical activity and incorporating practices like yoga can have profound effects on managing menopausal symptoms and promoting overall well-being. In this article, we explore the benefits of yoga and exercise during menopause, how they can support various aspects of health, and practical strategies for integrating these activities into a holistic approach to wellness.

•Understanding Menopause and Its Impact

Menopause is characterized by the cessation of menstruation and a decline in reproductive hormones, particularly estrogen and progesterone. This hormonal transition can lead to a variety of symptoms, including hot flashes, mood swings, weight gain, bone density loss, and more.

•The Power of Yoga for Menopause

Yoga and exercise can play a significant role in managing the symptoms of menopause. As women go through this natural transition, they often experience various physical and emotional changes, including hot flashes, mood swings, weight gain, and decreased bone density. Regular physical activity, including yoga, can help alleviate these symptoms and promote overall well-being.

Yoga is a mind-body practice that combines physical postures, breathing exercises, and meditation. It has been practiced for centuries and is known for its numerous health benefits. During menopause, yoga can be particularly beneficial in several ways.

Firstly, yoga helps to reduce hot flashes and night sweats, which are common symptoms of menopause. The gentle stretching and relaxation techniques in yoga help calm the nervous system and regulate body temperature. Additionally, deep breathing exercises can help manage stress and anxiety, which can contribute to the intensity and frequency of hot flashes.

Secondly, yoga promotes bone health. As estrogen levels decline during menopause, women become more susceptible to osteoporosis, a condition characterized by weak and brittle bones. Weight-bearing exercises, such as yoga, help increase bone density and reduce the risk of fractures. Poses like Downward Dog, Triangle, and Warrior II are particularly beneficial for strengthening the bones and muscles.

Thirdly, yoga improves flexibility and joint health. As women age, they may experience joint stiffness and reduced range of motion. Yoga poses gently stretch and lengthen the muscles,

improving flexibility and joint mobility. This can help alleviate joint pain and stiffness commonly associated with menopause.

Furthermore, yoga enhances mood and mental well-being. Menopause can bring about mood swings, irritability, and feelings of depression. The mindfulness and meditation aspects of yoga promote relaxation, reduce stress, and improve emotional balance. The release of endorphins during exercise also contributes to a positive mood and overall sense of well-being.

In addition to yoga, incorporating other forms of exercise into a menopausal woman's routine can provide further benefits. Aerobic exercises, such as brisk walking, swimming, or cycling, help maintain cardiovascular health and manage weight gain, which is a common concern during menopause. Strength training exercises, using resistance bands or weights, can help maintain muscle mass and prevent age-related muscle loss.

It's important to note that each woman's experience of menopause is unique, and it's essential to consult with a healthcare professional before starting any exercise program. They can provide personalized recommendations based on individual health conditions, fitness levels, and goals.

•Emotional and Mental Benefits of Yoga

1. Stress Reduction: Yoga promotes relaxation through breath awareness and meditation, reducing stress hormones and fostering emotional well-being.
2. Mood Enhancement: Yoga has been shown to increase levels of serotonin, a neurotransmitter associated with mood regulation.
3. Mindfulness: The meditative aspects of yoga cultivate mindfulness, helping individuals manage negative thought patterns and increase self-awareness.

4. Sleep Improvement: Practicing yoga regularly can lead to improved sleep quality by calming the mind and reducing anxiety.

•Selecting the Right Type of Yoga

1. Hatha Yoga: Gentle and suitable for all levels, Hatha yoga focuses on basic poses and breath control.
2. Vinyasa Yoga: A dynamic practice that flows through sequences of poses, Vinyasa yoga builds strength and flexibility.
3. Restorative Yoga: A deeply relaxing practice that uses props to support the body, restorative yoga is particularly helpful for stress reduction.
4. Yin Yoga: Slow-paced and focused on holding poses for extended periods, Yin yoga targets connective tissues and promotes flexibility.

•Practical Strategies for Incorporating Yoga

1. Set Realistic Goals: Start with a feasible commitment, gradually increasing the duration and intensity of your practice.
2. Practice Consistency: Dedicate a specific time for yoga practice each day or several times a week.
   *Listen to Your Body: Choose poses and sequences that align with your current physical condition. Modify or skip poses that feel uncomfortable.
3. Mindful Breathing: Integrate deep, mindful breathing into your practice to enhance relaxation and focus.
4. Guidance and Instruction: Attend yoga classes, watch instructional videos, or use yoga apps to learn proper alignment and techniques.

•Exercise for Menopause: Embracing Physical Vitality

Engaging in regular exercise, beyond yoga, is equally essential for managing menopausal symptoms and promoting overall health.

-Cardiovascular Exercise

1. Aerobic Activities: Walking, jogging, swimming, cycling, and dancing are effective for cardiovascular health.

2. Benefits: Cardiovascular exercise supports heart health, boosts mood, enhances metabolism, and aids weight management.

-Strength Training

1. Resistance Exercises: Incorporate weightlifting, bodyweight exercises, or resistance bands to strengthen muscles.
2. Benefits: Strength training maintains muscle mass, supports bone health, and contributes to overall vitality.

-Flexibility and Balance Training

1. Tai Chi: This mind-body practice combines flowing movements and deep breathing to enhance flexibility, balance, and relaxation.
2. Benefits: Improving flexibility and balance reduces the risk of falls and supports joint health.

•Customizing an Exercise Routine

1. Multifaceted Approach: A well-rounded routine combines cardiovascular exercise, strength training, flexibility training, and relaxation techniques.
2. Consult a Professional: Prior to starting an exercise regimen, consult a healthcare provider, especially if you have underlying health conditions.

•Holistic Approach to Wellness

1. Nutrition: Support your exercise routine with a balanced diet rich in nutrients that promote bone health, energy, and overall vitality.
2. Mindfulness: Incorporate mindfulness practices to manage stress and promote emotional well-being alongside physical activity.
3. Rest and Recovery: Ensure adequate rest and sleep to support muscle recovery and overall wellness.

Yoga and exercise offer potent tools for women navigating the intricate landscape of menopause. By embracing the physical and mental benefits of yoga, engaging in cardiovascular activities, strength training, and flexibility exercises, women can foster well-being, manage symptoms, and promote vitality during this transformative phase of life. A holistic approach that combines these practices with balanced nutrition, mindfulness, and self-care rituals empowers women to thrive during menopause, embracing the journey with strength, resilience, and an unwavering commitment to their overall health and wellness.

Chapter Five

Lifestyle Adjustments

Sleep Strategies

Menopause, a natural phase of life, brings about hormonal shifts that can impact various aspects of health, including sleep. Sleep disturbances are common during menopause, characterized by difficulties falling asleep, staying asleep, or experiencing restful sleep. Understanding the connection between menopause and sleep and adopting effective sleep strategies can greatly improve overall well-being. In this article, we delve into the challenges women face with sleep during menopause, explore the factors contributing to these disruptions, and provide practical strategies to promote restful nights.

•Sleep Challenges in Menopause

Sleep challenges are a common concern for women going through menopause. Hormonal fluctuations, hot flashes, night sweats, and other symptoms can disrupt sleep patterns and lead to insomnia or poor sleep quality. Understanding these sleep challenges and implementing strategies to improve sleep can significantly enhance the overall well-being of menopausal women.

One of the primary factors contributing to sleep disturbances during menopause is hormonal changes. As women approach menopause, their estrogen and progesterone levels decline. These hormones play a crucial role in regulating sleep patterns and promoting deep, restful sleep. The fluctuation and eventual decrease in these hormones can disrupt the body's natural sleep-wake cycle, leading to difficulties falling asleep or staying asleep throughout the night.

Hot flashes and night sweats are another common symptom of menopause that can interfere with sleep. These sudden episodes of intense heat and sweating can occur at any time, including during sleep. They can cause discomfort, awakenings, and difficulty returning to sleep, resulting in fragmented sleep and daytime fatigue.

Mood swings, anxiety, and stress are also prevalent during menopause and can contribute to sleep disturbances. The physical and emotional changes associated with this life stage can lead to racing thoughts, restlessness, and difficulty quieting the mind at bedtime. Additionally, the hormonal fluctuations can affect mood and exacerbate feelings of anxiety or depression, further impacting sleep quality.

•Promoting Sleep Hygiene: Creating a Sleep-Conducive Environment

1. Establish a Sleep Schedule: Go to bed and wake up at the same time every day, even on weekends, to regulate your body's internal clock.
2. Create a Comfortable Sleep Environment: Ensure your bedroom is dark, quiet, and at a comfortable temperature. Invest in a comfortable mattress and pillows.
3. Limit Screen Time: Reduce exposure to screens (phones, tablets, computers, TVs) before bedtime, as the blue light can interfere with sleep-inducing hormones.
4. Mindful Eating: Avoid heavy meals, caffeine, and alcohol close to bedtime. These substances can disrupt sleep and digestion.
5. Relaxation Rituals: Engage in calming activities before bed, such as reading, gentle stretching, or practicing deep breathing exercises.

•Managing Hot Flashes and Night Sweats

1. Layer Bedding: Use layers of bedding so you can easily adjust your covers during temperature fluctuations.

2. Breathable Fabrics: Opt for lightweight, breathable fabrics for your sleepwear and bedding to help regulate body temperature.
3. Cooling Pillows: Consider using pillows with cooling gel inserts to alleviate discomfort from hot flashes.

•Coping with Insomnia and Anxiety

1. Mindfulness Meditation: Engage in mindfulness meditation to calm racing thoughts and promote relaxation before bedtime.
2. Progressive Muscle Relaxation: This technique involves tensing and then relaxing each muscle group to release tension and promote relaxation.
3. Guided Imagery: Visualize calming and peaceful scenes to help shift your focus away from anxious thoughts.

•Addressing Restless Leg Syndrome

1. Regular Exercise: Engage in regular physical activity to help reduce restless leg symptoms.
2. Warm Baths: Soaking in a warm bath before bed can relax the muscles and alleviate discomfort.
3. Calf Stretches: Gentle stretches before bed can help reduce muscle tension and alleviate restless leg symptoms.

•Consulting a Healthcare Provider

1. Hormone Replacement Therapy (HRT): For some women, HRT may alleviate sleep disturbances by addressing hormonal imbalances. Consult a healthcare provider to discuss the benefits and risks.
2. Sleep Medications: If sleep disturbances are severe, short-term use of sleep medications may be considered under the guidance of a healthcare provider.

•Lifestyle Changes for Better Sleep

1. Regular Exercise: Engage in regular physical activity during the day, but avoid intense exercise close to bedtime.

2. Balanced Diet: Consume a well-balanced diet that includes foods rich in magnesium (e.g., nuts, seeds, leafy greens) and tryptophan (e.g., turkey, dairy, bananas), which support relaxation and sleep.
3. Limit Fluid Intake: Minimize fluid intake close to bedtime to reduce nighttime awakenings for bathroom trips.
4. Caffeine and Alcohol: Limit caffeine and alcohol intake, especially in the evening, as they can disrupt sleep.
5. Stress Management: Practice stress-reduction techniques such as yoga, meditation, and deep breathing exercises to calm the mind and promote relaxation.

Sleep disturbances during menopause are a common challenge, but they can be effectively managed with the right strategies and lifestyle changes. By adopting sleep hygiene practices, addressing specific symptoms like hot flashes and anxiety, and making thoughtful adjustments to your daily routine, you can significantly improve the quality of your sleep and overall well-being during this transformative phase. Remember that each woman's experience is unique, so it may take some trial and error to find the strategies that work best for you. With dedication and a proactive approach to sleep, you can navigate menopause with restful nights and wake up feeling refreshed and revitalized.

Maintaining Bone Health

Menopause is a natural phase in a woman's life marked by hormonal shifts that can have significant effects on bone health. As estrogen levels decline, the risk of bone loss and osteoporosis increases. Maintaining strong and healthy bones is essential to overall well-being and quality of life. In this article, we explore the impact of menopause on bone health, delve into the factors contributing to bone loss, and provide practical strategies for preserving bone density and promoting skeletal strength during this transformative phase.

•Understanding Bone Health and Menopause

During menopause, women experience significant changes in their hormone levels, particularly a decrease in estrogen. These hormonal changes can have a profound impact on bone health. Understanding the relationship between menopause and bone health is crucial for women to take proactive steps in maintaining strong and healthy bones.

Estrogen plays a vital role in maintaining bone density and strength. It helps regulate the balance between bone formation and bone resorption, the process of breaking down old bone tissue. When estrogen levels decline during menopause, this delicate balance is disrupted, leading to an increased rate of bone loss. This loss of bone density can eventually lead to osteoporosis, a condition characterized by weak and brittle bones that are more prone to fractures.

The years leading up to menopause, known as perimenopause, are particularly critical for bone health. During this time, estrogen levels fluctuate, and bone loss may accelerate. It is estimated that women can lose up to 20% of their bone density in the five to seven years following menopause.

•Factors Contributing to Bone Loss during Menopause

Several factors contribute to bone loss during menopause:

1. Hormonal Changes: Estrogen helps regulate bone remodeling by inhibiting bone resorption. As estrogen declines, bone resorption becomes more prevalent.
2. Age: Age-related factors also contribute to decreased bone density, making older women more susceptible to bone loss.
3. Nutritional Factors: Inadequate intake of calcium, vitamin D, and other bone-supportive nutrients can exacerbate bone loss.
4. Lifestyle Factors: Lack of weight-bearing exercise, smoking, excessive alcohol consumption, and certain medications can weaken bones.

•Strategies for Maintaining Bone Health

1. Calcium and Vitamin D Intake
   - Calcium: Calcium is a crucial mineral for bone health. Include dairy products, leafy greens, fortified foods, and calcium-rich plant-based options in your diet.
   - Vitamin D: Vitamin D enhances calcium absorption and promotes bone health. Exposure to sunlight, fortified foods, and supplements can provide sufficient vitamin D.
3. Weight-Bearing Exercise
   - Engaging in weight-bearing exercises like walking, jogging, dancing, and resistance training helps stimulate bone formation and strengthens bones.

4. Resistance Training
   - Weight lifting and resistance exercises help build bone density by putting stress on bones and promoting bone formation.
5. Balanced Diet
   - Consume a well-balanced diet rich in nutrients like magnesium, vitamin K, and vitamin C, which support bone health.
6. Reduce Alcohol and Smoking
   - Limit alcohol consumption and quit smoking to prevent bone loss and reduce fracture risk.
7. Hormone Replacement Therapy (HRT)
   - Consult a healthcare provider to discuss the benefits and risks of HRT, which may help preserve bone density by maintaining estrogen levels.
8. Calcium and Vitamin D Supplements
   - If dietary intake is insufficient, supplements can help meet calcium and vitamin D needs. Consult a healthcare provider before starting supplements.

•Bone-Boosting Nutrients and Foods

1. Calcium-Rich Foods
   - Dairy products (low-fat or non-fat options), fortified plant-based milk, leafy greens (kale, collard greens), almonds, and tofu.
2. Vitamin D-Rich Foods
   - Fatty fish (salmon, mackerel), fortified dairy or plant-based milk, eggs, and exposure to sunlight.
3. Magnesium-Rich Foods
   - Nuts (almonds, cashews), seeds (pumpkin seeds, sunflower seeds), whole grains, and leafy greens.
4. Vitamin K-Rich Foods
   - Leafy greens (spinach, kale, broccoli), Brussels sprouts, and fermented foods.

•Regular Physical Activity for Bone Health

1. Weight-Bearing Exercises
   - Walking, jogging, dancing, hiking, and stair climbing help stimulate bone formation.
2. Resistance Exercises
   - Weight lifting, bodyweight exercises, and resistance bands strengthen muscles and bones.
3. Yoga and Pilates

- These practices focus on balance, flexibility, and strength, contributing to overall bone health.

•Lifestyle Choices for Strong Bones

1. Maintain a Healthy Weight
   - Achieving and maintaining a healthy weight reduces the strain on bones and minimizes the risk of fractures.
2. Limit Caffeine and Salt Intake
   - Excessive caffeine and salt consumption can contribute to calcium loss. Moderation is key.
3. Stay Hydrated
   - Drinking enough water supports overall health, including bone health.

•Regular Bone Health Assessments

1. Bone Density Testing
   - Regular bone density tests (DEXA scans) can assess your bone health and help you track changes over time.
2. Consult a Healthcare Provider
   - Discuss your bone health with a healthcare provider, especially if you have risk factors or concerns about osteoporosis.

Preserving bone health during menopause requires a proactive approach that encompasses nutrition, exercise, and lifestyle choices. By focusing on adequate calcium and vitamin D intake, engaging in weight-bearing and resistance exercises, adopting a balanced diet rich in bone-boosting nutrients, and making thoughtful lifestyle choices, women can navigate the challenges of bone loss with resilience and grace. Prioritizing bone health during menopause ensures not only a strong foundation for physical activity but also contributes to overall vitality and quality of life.

Maintaining Heart Health

The decline in estrogen levels during menopause can influence cardiovascular risk factors and increase the risk of heart disease. However, with knowledge and proactive strategies, women can maintain and promote heart health during this stage of life. In this article, we delve into the impact of menopause on cardiovascular health, explore the factors contributing to cardiovascular risk, and provide practical strategies for promoting heart wellness and reducing the risk of heart disease.

•Understanding Menopause and Cardiovascular Health

Menopause marks the end of a woman's reproductive years and is defined by the cessation of menstruation for 12 consecutive months. This transition is primarily driven by a decline in estrogen production by the ovaries. Estrogen plays a protective role in cardiovascular health, influencing factors such as blood vessel function, cholesterol levels, and inflammation.

•Cardiovascular Changes during Menopause

The hormonal changes during menopause can contribute to several cardiovascular changes:

1. Increased Cardiovascular Risk: The decline in estrogen is associated with unfavorable changes in cholesterol profiles, increased inflammation, and changes in blood vessel function, all of which contribute to higher cardiovascular risk.
2. Changes in Cholesterol: Estrogen helps maintain a favorable balance of "good" (HDL) and "bad" (LDL) cholesterol. With its decline, LDL cholesterol levels can increase, contributing to atherosclerosis.
3. Blood Pressure: Estrogen helps relax blood vessels, contributing to normal blood pressure. Its decline can lead to stiffer blood vessels and higher blood pressure.
4. Insulin Sensitivity: Estrogen supports insulin sensitivity and glucose regulation. Lower estrogen levels can affect glucose metabolism.

•Reducing Cardiovascular Risk Factors

1. Healthy Diet
   - Embrace a diet rich in whole grains, fruits, vegetables, lean proteins, and healthy fats (e.g., olive oil, nuts, fatty fish).
   - Limit saturated and trans fats, added sugars, and sodium to reduce the risk of high blood pressure, high cholesterol, and weight gain.

2. Regular Physical Activity
   - Engage in at least 150 minutes of moderate-intensity aerobic activity or 75 minutes of vigorous-intensity activity per week.
   - Include strength training exercises to improve muscle mass and metabolism.
3. Maintain a Healthy Weight
   - Achieve and maintain a healthy weight to reduce the risk of cardiovascular disease and related risk factors.
4. Manage Stress

- Engage in stress-reducing activities such as meditation, deep breathing, yoga, and mindfulness to lower stress hormone levels and promote heart health.

•Addressing Specific Cardiovascular Risk Factors

1. Cholesterol Management
   - Monitor cholesterol levels and discuss treatment options with a healthcare provider if necessary.
   - Focus on dietary changes, exercise, and, if needed, medication to manage cholesterol levels.
2. Blood Pressure Control
   - Monitor blood pressure regularly and follow healthcare provider recommendations for maintaining healthy levels.
   - Lifestyle changes, including a balanced diet, exercise, stress reduction, and potential medication, can help control blood pressure.
3. Diabetes Prevention and Management
   - Maintain a healthy diet, engage in regular exercise, and monitor blood glucose levels to reduce the risk of diabetes.
   - If diagnosed with diabetes, work with healthcare providers to manage blood sugar levels through lifestyle changes and, if necessary, medication.
4. Quitting Smoking
   - Quit smoking to reduce the risk of heart disease and related complications.
   - Seek support through smoking cessation programs, counseling, and medication if needed.

•Hormone Replacement Therapy (HRT)

Hormone replacement therapy (HRT) has been a topic of interest in relation to cardiovascular health in menopause. Menopause is a natural stage in a woman's life when her menstrual periods cease, and hormone levels, particularly estrogen, decline. Estrogen plays a significant role in

maintaining cardiovascular health, and the decline in estrogen during menopause is associated with an increased risk of cardiovascular disease.

HRT involves the administration of hormones, typically estrogen and progesterone, to replace the declining levels. It can be given as estrogen-only therapy (ET) to women who have undergone a hysterectomy or as combined estrogen-progestogen therapy (EPT) to women who still have their uterus.

Several studies have investigated the impact of HRT on cardiovascular health in menopause. The findings have been mixed, and the benefits and risks of HRT should be carefully considered on an individual basis.

One of the potential benefits of HRT in cardiovascular health is its ability to improve lipid profiles. Estrogen has been shown to increase levels of high-density lipoprotein (HDL) cholesterol, often referred to as "good" cholesterol, which helps remove low-density lipoprotein (LDL) cholesterol, or "bad" cholesterol, from the arteries. This can contribute to a reduction in the risk of atherosclerosis, a condition characterized by the buildup of plaque in the arteries.

Additionally, estrogen has been found to have a positive impact on blood vessel function. It helps maintain the elasticity and integrity of blood vessels, promoting healthy blood flow and reducing the risk of hypertension (high blood pressure). Hypertension is a major risk factor for cardiovascular disease, including heart attacks and strokes.

However, it is important to note that the benefits of HRT on cardiovascular health may vary depending on factors such as the timing of initiation, duration of use, and individual characteristics. The Women's Health Initiative (WHI) study, a large-scale clinical trial, found that HRT use in postmenopausal women aged 50-79 years was associated with an increased risk of cardiovascular events, including heart attacks and strokes. These findings led to a decline in the use of HRT for cardiovascular health purposes.

It is crucial to consider the potential risks associated with HRT in cardiovascular health. The WHI study also reported an increased risk of blood clots, which can lead to deep vein thrombosis or pulmonary embolism. The risk of blood clots appears to be higher during the first year of HRT use and in women who have preexisting risk factors.

•Lifestyle Choices for Heart Health

1. Limit Alcohol Consumption
   - If you choose to drink, do so in moderation (up to one drink per day for women) to reduce the risk of heart disease.
2. Stay Hydrated
   - Drinking enough water supports overall health, including cardiovascular health.
3. Regular Check-Ups and Screenings
   - Schedule regular health check-ups and screenings to monitor blood pressure, cholesterol levels, and other cardiovascular risk factors.

Maintaining heart health during menopause requires a multifaceted approach that encompasses lifestyle changes, awareness of risk factors, and proactive management of cardiovascular health. By adopting a balanced diet, engaging in regular physical activity, managing stress, and addressing specific risk factors, women can navigate the hormonal changes of menopause with resilience and promote long-term heart wellness. Taking charge of heart health empowers women to embrace menopause with vitality, ensuring that this transformative phase of life is marked by cardiovascular well-being and an enduring commitment to overall health.

Chapter Six

Creating a Supportive Environment

Communication with Loved Ones

Effective communication with loved ones during this phase can play a vital role in maintaining relationships, fostering understanding, and navigating the emotional and physical changes that come with menopause. In this article, we delve into the importance of open communication during menopause, explore the challenges that can arise, and provide practical strategies for nurturing connections and fostering mutual support among family members, partners, and friends.

•The Importance of Communication during Menopause

Effective communication during menopause is crucial for maintaining healthy relationships, managing symptoms, and seeking support. Menopause is a natural biological process that marks the end of a woman's reproductive years. It is accompanied by various physical and emotional changes due to hormonal fluctuations.

Open and honest communication with loved ones, including partners, family, and friends, is essential during this time. Menopause can bring about mood swings, irritability, and changes in libido, which can impact relationships. By openly discussing these changes, both partners can better understand and support each other.

Communication is also vital in seeking support from healthcare professionals. Menopause symptoms can vary greatly from woman to woman, and discussing them with a trusted healthcare provider can help in finding appropriate treatments or lifestyle changes to manage symptoms effectively.

Additionally, communication with healthcare providers can help in addressing any concerns or questions about hormone replacement therapy (HRT) or other treatment options. By discussing the potential benefits and risks, women can make informed decisions about their healthcare during menopause.

Communication is not limited to verbal exchanges. Non-verbal cues, such as body language and facial expressions, can also convey emotions and needs. Partners and loved ones should be attentive to these cues and provide support and understanding.

In addition to interpersonal communication, self-communication is crucial during menopause. This involves being aware of one's own feelings, needs, and boundaries. By practicing self-reflection and self-care, women can better manage their emotional well-being and communicate their needs effectively to others.

Support groups and online communities can also provide a platform for communication and sharing experiences with other women going through menopause. These interactions can offer validation, advice, and a sense of community, helping women navigate through this transitional phase.

Lastly, communication with oneself is important during menopause. This involves acknowledging and accepting the changes happening in the body and mind. By practicing self-compassion and self-acceptance, women can embrace this new phase of life with confidence and resilience.

In summary, effective communication during menopause is crucial for maintaining healthy relationships, seeking support, and managing symptoms. Open and honest discussions with loved ones and healthcare providers can foster understanding and provide the necessary support. Additionally, self-communication and self-acceptance play a vital role in navigating through this transformative phase of life.

•Challenges in Communication during Menopause

1. Emotional Changes: Hormonal fluctuations can lead to mood swings, irritability, and emotional sensitivity, which may impact interactions with loved ones.
2. Physical Discomfort: Symptoms like hot flashes, sleep disturbances, and fatigue can affect daily routines and communication patterns.
3. Self-Identity: Menopause can trigger reflections on identity and aging, leading to changes in self-perception and potentially affecting communication.

•Strategies for Effective Communication

1. Open and Honest Dialogue
   - Encourage open conversations about menopause, sharing thoughts, feelings, and experiences with loved ones.
   - Create a safe space where everyone feels comfortable expressing their concerns and questions.
2. Educate and Raise Awareness
   - Provide information about menopause to loved ones, enabling them to better understand the physical and emotional changes you're experiencing.
   - Share resources, articles, or books that offer insights into menopause and its impact.
3. Expressing Needs and Boundaries
   - Clearly communicate your needs, whether it's alone time, emotional support, or specific adjustments to daily routines.

- Establish healthy boundaries that respect both your needs and those of your loved
  ones.
4. Empathy and Active Listening
   - Practice active listening when loved ones share their thoughts and concerns.
   - Show empathy by acknowledging their feelings and validating their experiences.
5. Managing Conflict
   - If conflicts arise, approach them with patience and a willingness to understand
     each other's perspectives.
   - Focus on resolving issues through compromise and open dialogue rather than
     escalating disagreements.

•Support from Partners

1. Mutual Understanding
   - Partners should actively seek to understand the physical and emotional changes
     associated with menopause.
   - Offer patience and empathy while listening to concerns and experiences.
2. Emotional Support
   - Provide emotional support and reassurance, recognizing that menopause can be a
     challenging time emotionally.
   - Offer comfort during times of mood swings or irritability, without judgment.
3. Participate in Lifestyle Changes
   - Engage in healthy lifestyle changes together, such as adopting a balanced diet,
     regular exercise, and stress reduction practices.
   - Encourage and support each other's efforts to prioritize well-being.

•Family and Friends

1. Education and Awareness
   - Educate family members and friends about menopause to foster understanding
     and empathy.
   - Share how menopause can impact daily life and why certain adjustments are
     necessary.
2. Engage in Dialogue
   - Maintain open lines of communication about how menopause may affect your
     interactions.
   - Encourage family members and friends to express their thoughts and concerns as
     well.

3. Celebrate Achievements
    - Share your triumphs and accomplishments, celebrating the positive aspects of navigating menopause.
    - Encourage loved ones to recognize and celebrate your resilience and growth.

•Children and Teens

1. Age-Appropriate Discussions
    - Approach discussions about menopause with children and teens based on their age and understanding.
    - Provide simple explanations that help them grasp the changes you're experiencing.
2. Modeling Communication
    - Demonstrate healthy communication skills by engaging in open conversations with your children and teens.
    - Emphasize the importance of expressing feelings, asking questions, and offering support.

Navigating menopause is a journey that not only affects the individual experiencing it but also their loved ones. Effective communication during this phase is essential for maintaining strong relationships, fostering understanding, and creating an environment of empathy and support. By embracing open dialogue, educating loved ones about menopause, expressing needs and boundaries, and practicing active listening, individuals can navigate the challenges of menopause while nurturing connections with partners, family, and friends. Through compassionate communication, both individuals and their loved ones can navigate this transformative phase with grace, empathy, and a deepened bond that strengthens the fabric of relationships.

Seeking Professional Guidance

While menopause is a universal experience, each woman's journey is unique, and seeking professional guidance during this time can provide invaluable support, guidance, and personalized care. In this article, we delve into the significance of seeking professional guidance during menopause, explore the types of healthcare providers who can offer assistance, and provide practical insights into the comprehensive care available to women as they navigate this transformative life stage.

•Understanding the Need for Professional Guidance

Menopause encompasses a range of physical and emotional changes that can significantly impact a woman's quality of life. From managing symptoms such as hot flashes, mood swings, and sleep disturbances to addressing long-term health considerations like bone density and cardiovascular health, seeking professional guidance ensures that women receive accurate information, personalized care, and evidence-based interventions tailored to their unique needs.

•Types of Healthcare Providers

1. Primary Care Physicians
   - Primary care physicians play a crucial role in managing overall health and coordinating care during menopause.
   - They can provide guidance on lifestyle modifications, address common symptoms, and monitor general health.
2. Gynecologists
   - Gynecologists specialize in women's reproductive health and can offer expert guidance on menopausal symptoms, hormone replacement therapy (HRT), and more.
   - They can perform regular check-ups, screenings, and preventive care specific to women's health.
3. Endocrinologists
   - Endocrinologists specialize in hormonal imbalances and can provide comprehensive care for managing hormonal changes during menopause.
   - They may offer guidance on hormonal therapies and manage conditions like thyroid disorders that can influence menopausal symptoms.
4. Cardiologists
   - Cardiologists specialize in heart health and can provide insights into maintaining cardiovascular well-being during and after menopause.
   - They can assess risk factors and recommend lifestyle changes to promote heart health.
5. Mental Health Professionals
   - Mental health professionals, including psychologists and therapists, can offer support for managing emotional changes and mood swings during menopause.
   - They can provide coping strategies and interventions to address anxiety, depression, and other emotional challenges.
6. Nutritionists/Dietitians
   - Nutritionists and dietitians can provide guidance on maintaining a balanced diet to support overall health and manage symptoms during menopause.

- They can offer personalized nutritional recommendations based on individual needs and goals.

7. Physical Therapists
   - Physical therapists can assist in managing musculoskeletal changes and address any physical challenges associated with menopause.
   - They can provide exercises and techniques to improve flexibility, strength, and mobility.

•Benefits of Seeking Professional Guidance

1. Accurate Information
   - Healthcare providers offer evidence-based information about menopause, dispelling myths and providing accurate insights.
2. Personalized Care
   - Professionals tailor care to individual needs, considering factors such as medical history, lifestyle, and specific symptoms.
3. Symptom Management
   - Healthcare providers offer strategies and interventions to manage common symptoms like hot flashes, sleep disturbances, and mood swings.
4. Preventive Health
   - Professionals can assess and address risk factors for conditions like osteoporosis, cardiovascular disease, and more.
5. Hormone Replacement Therapy (HRT)
   - When appropriate, healthcare providers can discuss the benefits and risks of HRT for managing menopausal symptoms.
6. Emotional Support
   - Mental health professionals provide a safe space to discuss emotional challenges and offer coping strategies.

•Preparing for Professional Visits

1. Compile Information
   - Make a list of symptoms, questions, and concerns to discuss during appointments.
2. Health History
   - Share your medical history, including any preexisting conditions, medications, and family history.
3. Open Communication

- Be open and honest about your experiences, concerns, and goals with healthcare providers.
4. Ask Questions
    - Don't hesitate to ask questions about treatment options, potential side effects, and long-term health considerations.

5. Take Notes
    - Keep notes from appointments to track recommendations, interventions, and changes in your health.

Seeking professional guidance during menopause is a proactive and empowering step toward achieving optimal health and well-being. Healthcare providers play a pivotal role in offering accurate information, personalized care, and evidence-based interventions that address the unique challenges of menopause. By collaborating with primary care physicians, gynecologists, endocrinologists, mental health professionals, and other experts, women can navigate the physical, emotional, and psychological changes of menopause with confidence, resilience, and a comprehensive support system. Embracing professional guidance ensures that women not only manage the challenges of menopause effectively but also thrive and enjoy this transformative phase of life to the fullest.

Joining Menopause Support Groups

Menopause significant that it can bring about a range of physical, emotional, and psychological changes. Navigating these changes can sometimes be challenging, but the journey doesn't have to be taken alone. Joining menopause support groups can provide women with a valuable source of connection, empathy, and empowerment. In this article, we explore the benefits of joining menopause support groups, delve into the types of groups available, and offer practical insights into how these groups can enhance well-being during this transformative phase.

•The Power of Connection and Support

Menopause is a shared experience that millions of women go through, yet it's often experienced in isolation. Joining a support group offers the opportunity to connect with others who are going through similar challenges, creating a sense of camaraderie and understanding that can be deeply comforting.

•Benefits of Joining Menopause Support Groups

1. Validation and Understanding
    - Support groups provide a space where women can share their experiences and feelings without judgment.

    - Being understood and validated by others who are facing similar challenges can reduce feelings of isolation and loneliness.
2. Empowerment and Knowledge
    - Support groups offer a platform for sharing information, resources, and strategies for managing menopause-related symptoms.
    - Women can empower themselves with knowledge about treatment options, lifestyle changes, and self-care practices.
3. Emotional Healing
    - Expressing feelings, fears, and concerns within a supportive environment can promote emotional healing and resilience.
    - Support group members often report feeling lighter and less burdened after sharing their thoughts and emotions.
4. Reduced Anxiety and Stress
    - Connecting with others who understand the journey can alleviate anxiety and stress associated with the uncertainties of menopause.
    - Sharing coping strategies can provide practical tools for managing stress and anxiety.
5. Sense of Community
    - Support groups foster a sense of belonging and community, which can boost overall well-being.
    - Building relationships with others in similar situations can lead to lasting friendships.
6. Shared Wisdom
    - Members can share personal insights and wisdom gained from their own journeys, offering valuable perspectives to others.
    - Learning from others' experiences can help members make informed decisions about their own health and well-being.

•Types of Menopause Support Groups

1. Local In-Person Groups
    - Local community centers, health clinics, and women's organizations often host in-person support groups.

- Meeting face-to-face allows for immediate connection and the opportunity to build strong, local friendships.

2. Online Support Groups
   - Online support groups provide a platform for women to connect virtually, regardless of geographical location.
   - These groups can offer a safe and convenient space for sharing experiences and seeking advice.

3. Specialized Support Groups
   - Some support groups cater to specific needs, such as those focusing on specific symptoms, lifestyle changes, or treatment options.
   - Specialized groups provide tailored information and insights related to specific concerns.

4. Peer-Led and Professional-Led Groups
   - Peer-led groups are facilitated by members who have personal experience with menopause.
   - Professional-led groups are led by healthcare providers, therapists, or specialists in menopause-related fields.
   -

•Participation Tips for Menopause Support Groups

1. Research and Choose Wisely
   - Explore different support groups to find one that aligns with your needs and preferences.
   - Consider factors such as meeting format, group size, and facilitator expertise.

2. Openness and Authenticity
   - Be open to sharing your thoughts, feelings, and experiences within the group.
   - Authenticity fosters deeper connections and promotes meaningful discussions.

3. Active Listening
   - Practice active listening when other members share their experiences.
   - Offer empathy and validation, creating a supportive atmosphere.

4. Respect and Confidentiality
   - Respect the privacy of others by maintaining confidentiality within the group.
   - Create a safe space where members feel comfortable sharing without fear of judgment.

5. Consistency and Commitment
   - Regular participation allows you to build stronger connections with group members.
   - Commit to attending meetings and engaging with the group.

Joining menopause support groups can be a transformative step toward navigating this life transition with strength, resilience, and a sense of community. The benefits of connecting with others who understand the challenges of menopause extend beyond emotional support—they encompass empowerment, shared knowledge, reduced stress, and a sense of belonging. Whether through local in-person groups, online communities, or specialized gatherings, women have the opportunity to create connections that empower them to embrace menopause with grace and confidence. By taking advantage of the collective wisdom and support available through menopause support groups, women can navigate this transformative phase with a renewed sense of empowerment, understanding, and optimism.

Chapter Seven
Embracing Change

Cultivating a Positive Outlook

Menopause is a natural and transformative phase in a woman's life that marks the end of the reproductive years. While it brings about hormonal changes and physical adjustments, it also presents an opportunity for personal growth, self-discovery, and empowerment. Cultivating a positive outlook during menopause can greatly influence one's experience, influencing not only physical well-being but also emotional resilience and overall quality of life. In this article, we delve into the importance of maintaining a positive perspective during menopause, explore strategies for cultivating positivity, and offer insights into how embracing change with optimism can lead to a fulfilling and enriching journey.

•The Power of a Positive Outlook

A positive outlook is a mindset that involves focusing on the potential for growth, embracing challenges, and finding the silver lining even in the midst of change. During menopause, a positive perspective can shape the way women navigate the transition, enabling them to make the most of this transformative phase.

•Benefits of Cultivating Positivity during Menopause

1. Emotional Resilience
    - A positive outlook enhances emotional resilience, enabling individuals to cope effectively with the emotional changes that may accompany menopause.

- A resilient mindset helps individuals bounce back from challenges, minimizing the impact of mood swings and emotional fluctuations.

2. Reduced Stress and Anxiety
   - Cultivating positivity lowers stress levels and reduces anxiety, contributing to overall emotional well-being.
   - A positive approach encourages individuals to manage stressors with a sense of calm and optimism.

3. Enhanced Coping Strategies
   - A positive perspective encourages the development of effective coping strategies to manage menopausal symptoms and challenges.
   - Individuals are more likely to seek and adopt healthy lifestyle changes when they approach them with a positive mindset.

4. Improved Physical Health
   - Studies have shown that a positive attitude can have a positive impact on physical health, potentially leading to better outcomes in managing symptoms like hot flashes and sleep disturbances.
   - A proactive attitude toward health encourages individuals to prioritize exercise, nutrition, and self-care.

5. Enhanced Relationships
   - A positive outlook fosters healthier interpersonal relationships by encouraging open communication and empathy.
   - Embracing change with positivity can lead to more supportive interactions with loved ones.

•Strategies for Cultivating Positivity during Menopause

1. Practice Gratitude
   - Regularly take time to reflect on the things you're grateful for, no matter how small.
   - Gratitude shifts focus away from challenges and cultivates a positive perspective.

2. Mindfulness and Meditation
   - Mindfulness practices and meditation help individuals stay present and centered, reducing stress and promoting emotional well-being.
   - These practices encourage a non-judgmental attitude toward one's thoughts and emotions.

3. Positive Affirmations
   - Use positive affirmations to reframe negative thoughts and beliefs.
   - Repeating affirmations like "I am resilient" or "I embrace change with grace" can shift your mindset over time.

4. Engage in Activities You Enjoy
    - Participate in hobbies and activities that bring joy and fulfillment.
    - Engaging in enjoyable pursuits boosts mood and contributes to a positive outlook.
5. Surround Yourself with Positivity*
    - Surround yourself with supportive friends and loved ones who uplift your spirits.
    - Minimize exposure to negativity, whether it's through media or toxic relationships.
6. Set Realistic Goals
    - Set achievable goals that align with your values and aspirations.
    - Accomplishing these goals boosts self-esteem and reinforces a positive outlook.

•Embracing Change with Optimism

1. View Change as Growth
    - Embrace menopause as an opportunity for personal growth, self-discovery, and empowerment.
    - Frame challenges as stepping stones toward a more fulfilling future.
2. Focus on the Present
    - Cultivate mindfulness by focusing on the present moment rather than dwelling on past regrets or future worries.
    - Embrace each day as a new chance to make positive choices.
3. Reframe Negative Thoughts
    - Challenge negative self-talk and reframe it with a more positive and compassionate perspective.
    - Instead of dwelling on limitations, focus on your strengths and potential.
    -

•Maintaining a Supportive Environment

1. Seek Supportive Relationships
    - Surround yourself with individuals who uplift your spirits and encourage a positive outlook.
    - Share your goals for cultivating positivity with loved ones, so they can provide encouragement.
2. Join Supportive Communities
    - Join menopause support groups or online communities where individuals share insights, challenges, and successes.
    - Connect with others who are embracing menopause with positivity.

Cultivating a positive outlook during menopause is a powerful choice that can significantly impact one's experience of this transformative phase. By embracing change with optimism, practicing gratitude, engaging in mindfulness, and surrounding yourself with positivity, you can navigate the challenges of menopause with resilience, emotional well-being, and a sense of empowerment. A positive perspective not only enhances your physical and emotional health but also enriches your relationships, personal growth, and overall quality of life. As you embrace menopause with a hopeful and open heart, you're setting the stage for a fulfilling and vibrant journey of self-discovery and renewal.

Rediscovering Passion and Purpose

Menopause is a natural and transformative phase that marks the end of a woman's reproductive years. While it brings about hormonal changes and physical adjustments, it also presents an opportunity for rediscovery and renewal. Rediscovering passion and purpose during menopause can be a transformative journey, leading to personal growth, self-fulfillment, and a renewed sense of vitality. In this article, we explore the importance of embracing this phase as a chance for rekindling passions and finding new purpose, delve into strategies for rediscovery, and offer insights into how embracing change can lead to a more enriching and fulfilling life.

•The Call for Rediscovery

Menopause signifies the closing of one chapter and the opening of another. As women transition from their reproductive years into a new phase of life, there's an opportunity to reevaluate goals, dreams, and desires. Rediscovering passion and purpose can invigorate this journey and infuse it with vitality.

•The Significance of Passion and Purpose

Passion refers to a strong, intense emotion, enthusiasm, or interest in an activity, subject, or pursuit. Purpose, on the other hand, relates to a sense of direction, meaning, and intention in life.

Both passion and purpose are integral to overall well-being, contributing to mental, emotional, and psychological health.

•Benefits of Rediscovering Passion and Purpose during Menopause

1. Enhanced Emotional Well-Being
   - Reconnecting with passions and finding new purpose brings joy, contentment, and a sense of fulfillment.
   - Engaging in activities that bring pleasure boosts mood and emotional well-being.
2. Stress Reduction
   - Immersing oneself in passions and purposeful pursuits can reduce stress levels and promote relaxation.
   - Engaging in activities that bring joy provides a natural outlet for releasing tension.
3. Increased Vitality
   - Rediscovering passion and purpose can infuse life with renewed energy and enthusiasm.
   - Pursuing interests and goals leads to a sense of vitality and zest for life.

4. Enhanced Self-Esteem
   - Accomplishing goals and engaging in meaningful activities boosts self-esteem and self-worth.
   - Rediscovery reinforces a positive self-image and confidence.
5. Sense of Accomplishment
   - Achieving personal goals, no matter how small, contributes to a sense of accomplishment and fulfillment.
   - Rediscovery fosters a sense of pride and a willingness to embrace new challenges.

•Strategies for Rediscovery

1. Reflect on Passions
   - Take time to reflect on past and current passions. What activities or interests bring you joy and excitement?
   - Reconnect with hobbies or pursuits that may have taken a backseat during the demands of daily life.
2. Explore New Interests
   - Use menopause as an opportunity to explore new hobbies or interests that have always intrigued you.
   - Attend classes, workshops, or events related to your newfound interests.
3. Prioritize Self-Care

    - Self-care activities, such as exercise, meditation, and relaxation techniques, contribute to overall well-being.
    - Self-care nourishes the mind, body, and soul, creating space for rediscovery.
4. Set Meaningful Goals
    - Identify short-term and long-term goals that align with your passions and desires.
    - Goal-setting provides direction and motivation for pursuing your interests.
5. Step Out of Your Comfort Zone
    - Embrace new challenges and experiences that push you beyond your comfort zone.
    - Stepping out of your comfort zone leads to personal growth and a sense of accomplishment.

•Finding New Purpose

1. Reflect on Values and Beliefs
    - Consider your core values, beliefs, and principles. What matters most to you?
    - Identifying your values can guide you toward activities and pursuits that align with your sense of purpose.

2. Contribute to Others
    - Volunteering or engaging in activities that benefit others can provide a sense of purpose and fulfillment.
    - Helping others fosters a sense of connection and makes a positive impact.
3. Lifelong Learning
    - Lifelong learning through classes, workshops, and online courses keeps the mind engaged and curious.
    - Learning new skills or expanding your knowledge contributes to personal growth and purpose.

•Embracing Change and Growth

1. Positive Mindset
    - Embrace change with a positive mindset, viewing it as an opportunity for growth and self-discovery.
    - A positive attitude enhances adaptability and resilience.
2. Stay Open to New Experiences
    - Be open to trying new things and exploring uncharted territories.

- New experiences can lead to unexpected passions and opportunities.
   3. Celebrate Small Wins
      - Celebrate every step forward, no matter how small. Each achievement contributes to your overall journey.
      - Small wins build momentum and encourage continued rediscovery.

Menopause is a pivotal phase that invites women to rediscover their passions and find new purpose, ultimately leading to a more fulfilling and enriched life. By reflecting on personal interests, setting meaningful goals, stepping out of comfort zones, and embracing change with optimism, women can embark on a transformative journey of self-discovery and renewal. Rekindling the flame of passion and purpose not only enhances emotional well-being and vitality but also reinforces self-esteem, resilience, and a positive outlook. Embracing menopause as an opportunity for rediscovery empowers women to navigate this transition with grace, enthusiasm, and a renewed sense of purpose that transcends the challenges and ushers in a new chapter of personal growth and fulfillment.

Embracing the Wisdom of Menopause

Menopause is a profound life transition that signals the end of a woman's reproductive years. While it brings about physical and hormonal changes, it also marks a gateway to a new phase of life—one that is rich with potential for growth, self-discovery, and wisdom. Embracing the wisdom of menopause involves recognizing the insights and lessons that come with this transformative experience. In this article, we explore the concept of embracing menopause as a source of wisdom, delve into the lessons it offers, and provide practical insights into how to tap into the transformative power of this life transition.

•Menopause as a Source of Wisdom

Menopause is not just a biological process; it is a transformative journey that can bring about a wealth of wisdom and self-discovery. As women transition from their reproductive years to a new phase of life, they often experience a range of physical and emotional changes. While these changes can be challenging, they also offer an opportunity for growth and self-reflection.

One of the ways menopause can be a source of wisdom is by prompting women to reevaluate their priorities and values. As the body undergoes hormonal changes, women may find themselves reassessing what truly matters to them. This may involve letting go of societal expectations or redefining their roles and identities. Menopause can be a catalyst for self-discovery and a chance to align one's life with their authentic desires and aspirations.

Menopause can also be a time of heightened self-awareness. The physical symptoms and emotional fluctuations that accompany this phase can serve as a reminder to prioritize self-care and listen to the body's needs. Women may become more attuned to their physical, emotional, and mental well-being, and make conscious choices to nurture themselves. This increased self-awareness can lead to a deeper understanding of one's own strengths, limitations, and boundaries.

Another aspect of menopause as a source of wisdom is the opportunity for personal growth and resilience. The challenges that come with this transition can be seen as opportunities for growth and adaptation. Women learn to navigate through physical discomfort, mood swings, and other symptoms, developing resilience and coping strategies along the way. This resilience can extend beyond menopause, empowering women to face future challenges with strength and grace.

Menopause can also provide a unique perspective on aging and mortality. As women enter this phase, they may confront their own mortality and reflect on the passage of time. This reflection can inspire a deeper appreciation for life and a sense of urgency to make the most of each day. Menopause can be a reminder to live fully, embrace new experiences, and cherish the relationships and moments that bring joy and fulfillment.

Furthermore, menopause can foster a sense of solidarity and connection among women. By openly discussing their experiences and supporting one another, women can create a community of shared wisdom. This collective knowledge can be a powerful resource for navigating through menopause and beyond. Women can learn from each other's stories, gain insights, and find comfort in knowing that they are not alone in their journey.

Menopause also offers an opportunity to redefine beauty and self-image. Society often places emphasis on youth and fertility, but menopause challenges these narrow definitions.

•The Lessons of Menopause

1. Self-Discovery
   - Menopause prompts self-reflection and introspection, encouraging women to examine their desires, values, and aspirations.
   - It's a time to reassess goals, embrace newfound interests, and honor the journey that led to this point.

2. Resilience and Adaptability
    - Menopause is a testament to the body's ability to adapt and change.
    - Embracing the physical changes associated with menopause can foster a greater sense of resilience and an acceptance of the body's natural evolution.
3. Navigating Change
    - Menopause teaches the importance of navigating change with grace and resilience.
    - By embracing change as a constant in life, women can develop adaptable mindsets that serve them in various situations.
4. Mind-Body Connection
    - Menopause emphasizes the interplay between physical health and emotional well-being.
    - Understanding the mind-body connection encourages holistic self-care and nurtures emotional resilience.

•Practical Strategies for Embracing the Wisdom of Menopause

1. Cultivate Mindfulness
    - Mindfulness practices, such as meditation and deep breathing, cultivate self-awareness and a deeper connection to inner wisdom.
    - Mindfulness helps women stay present, manage stress, and navigate emotions with greater clarity.
2. Journaling for Reflection
    - Keeping a journal allows women to reflect on their experiences, insights, and personal growth during menopause.

    - Writing provides a space for processing emotions and capturing moments of wisdom.
3. Engage in Self-Care Rituals
    - Self-care rituals, such as baths, walks in nature, or practicing hobbies, nurture the soul and encourage self-discovery.
    - Regular self-care routines create space for introspection and self-compassion.
4. Seek Knowledge
    - Educate yourself about menopause and the changes it brings. Understanding the physical and emotional shifts can empower you to embrace them more fully.
    - Knowledge is a cornerstone of wisdom, and learning about menopause can foster a greater sense of empowerment.

- # The Role of Resilience and Acceptance

    1. Embrace the Journey
        - Cultivate an attitude of acceptance toward the changes of menopause.
        - Embracing the journey with an open heart allows for a deeper connection to its transformative power.
    2. Adapt to Change
        - Approach physical changes with adaptability and a sense of grace.
        - Adapting to change fosters a greater sense of resilience, which can extend to various aspects of life.

- # Fostering Emotional Well-Being

    1. Practice Emotional Intelligence
        - Develop emotional intelligence by acknowledging and processing emotions as they arise.
        - Embracing emotions and seeking understanding can lead to greater emotional wisdom.
    2. Release Perfectionism
        - Embrace imperfections and let go of unrealistic expectations.
        - Recognize that wisdom comes from acknowledging mistakes and learning from them.

- # The Gift of Perspective

    1. Reflect on Life's Journey
        - Reflect on your life's journey, acknowledging the challenges, triumphs, and moments of growth.
        - A broader perspective can reveal the wisdom gained from navigating life's experiences.
    2. Share Wisdom with Others
        - Share the insights you've gained during menopause with others, whether through mentoring, writing, or conversations.
        - Sharing your wisdom can create connections and inspire others on their journeys.

Embracing the wisdom of menopause is an invitation to journey within, to explore the depths of self-awareness, and to extract insights from the transformative experience. Through self-discovery, resilience, and a willingness to adapt, women can tap into a wellspring of wisdom that extends beyond the physical changes of menopause. By cultivating mindfulness, practicing self-care, and embracing emotions, women can nurture emotional well-being and connect to their inner reservoir of wisdom. Ultimately, menopause is an opportunity to embrace change, adapt with grace, and emerge as wiser, more empowered individuals. As women embrace the wisdom of menopause, they illuminate a path for themselves and others—a path that leads to greater self-awareness, personal growth, and an enriched understanding of the complexities of life.

Chapter Eight

Recipes for Wellbeing

Nutrient-Rich Meal Ideas

Menopause is a natural phase in a woman's life that brings about hormonal changes and shifts in metabolism. Proper nutrition plays a crucial role in managing the symptoms and supporting overall health during this transitional period. Incorporating nutrient-rich foods into your meals can help alleviate symptoms, boost energy levels, and promote well-being. In this article, we'll explore the importance of nutrition during menopause, delve into key nutrients to focus on, and provide practical, delicious meal ideas to nourish your body during this transformative phase.

•The Role of Nutrition in Menopause

Nutrition plays a crucial role in supporting women during the menopausal transition. As the body goes through hormonal changes, maintaining a healthy diet can help alleviate symptoms, support overall well-being, and promote long-term health. Here are some key ways nutrition can positively impact menopause:

1. Managing weight: Menopause can bring about changes in metabolism and hormonal fluctuations that may lead to weight gain. A balanced diet rich in fruits, vegetables, whole grains, lean proteins, and healthy fats can help manage weight by providing essential nutrients while keeping calorie intake in check. It is important to focus on portion control and avoid excessive consumption of processed foods, sugary snacks, and beverages.
2. Supporting bone health: Estrogen plays a critical role in maintaining bone density, and its decline during menopause increases the risk of osteoporosis. Adequate calcium and vitamin D intake is essential for maintaining strong bones. Good sources of calcium include dairy products, leafy greens, and fortified foods. Vitamin D can be obtained from sunlight exposure or through dietary sources like fatty fish, egg yolks, and fortified products.
3. Reducing hot flashes: Hot flashes are a common symptom of menopause that can disrupt sleep and daily activities. Certain foods and beverages may trigger or exacerbate hot flashes, such as caffeine, alcohol, spicy foods, and hot beverages. It can be helpful to identify and avoid these triggers. Additionally, incorporating foods rich in phytoestrogens, such as soy products, flaxseeds, and legumes, may help reduce the frequency and intensity of hot flashes.
4. Supporting heart health: Estrogen has a protective effect on cardiovascular health, and its decline during menopause increases the risk of heart disease. A heart-healthy diet that is low in saturated and trans fats, cholesterol, and sodium, and rich in fruits, vegetables, whole grains, lean proteins, and healthy fats can help support cardiovascular health. Including omega-3 fatty acids from sources like fatty fish, flaxseeds, and walnuts can also be beneficial.
5. Managing mood swings and depression: Hormonal changes during menopause can contribute to mood swings and an increased risk of depression. A nutrient-rich diet that includes foods high in omega-3 fatty acids, B vitamins, and antioxidants can support mental well-being. Examples include fatty fish, leafy greens, whole grains, nuts, seeds, and berries. Additionally, staying hydrated and avoiding excessive caffeine and alcohol intake can help stabilize mood.

6. Supporting brain health: Cognitive changes, including memory lapses during menopause, can be challenging. A nutritious diet can play a role in supporting brain health. Consuming foods rich in antioxidants, such as berries, dark chocolate, and leafy greens, can help protect brain cells from oxidative stress. Including omega-3 fatty acids from sources like fatty fish, chia seeds, and walnuts may also support cognitive function.
7. Promoting overall well-being: Menopause is a time of transition that can bring physical and emotional changes. Eating a well-balanced diet can provide the necessary nutrients to support overall well-being. Including a variety of colorful fruits and vegetables, whole grains, lean proteins, and healthy fats can help provide essential vitamins, minerals, and antioxidants. Staying hydrated by drinking an adequate amount of water throughout the day is also important.

Remember, it's always best to consult with a healthcare professional or registered dietitian for personalized advice and recommendations tailored to your specific needs during menopause.

•Key Nutrients to Focus On

1. Calcium and Vitamin D

- Essential for maintaining bone health and preventing osteoporosis.

- Sources: Dairy products, fortified plant-based milk, leafy greens, fatty fish, and fortified cereals.

2. Omega-3 Fatty Acids

- Support heart health, cognitive function, and mood stability.

- Sources: Fatty fish (salmon, mackerel, sardines), flaxseeds, chia seeds, walnuts, and hemp seeds.

3. Fiber

- Promotes digestive health, helps with weight management, and stabilizes blood sugar levels.

- Sources: Whole grains, legumes, fruits, vegetables, nuts, and seeds.

4. Phytoestrogens

- Natural compounds that can help alleviate menopausal symptoms by mimicking estrogen in the body.

- Sources: Soy products (tofu, tempeh, edamame), flaxseeds, sesame seeds, and whole grains.

5. Antioxidants (Vitamins A, C, E)

- Protect cells from oxidative stress, boost immunity, and support skin health.

- Sources: Colorful fruits and vegetables (berries, citrus fruits, bell peppers, spinach), nuts, and seeds.

6. Iron and Vitamin B12

- Important for maintaining energy levels and preventing anemia.

- Sources: Lean meats, poultry, fish, fortified plant-based foods, leafy greens, and lentils.

•Nutrient-Rich Meal Ideas

1. Breakfast Options

a. Berry and Yogurt Parfait:

  - Greek yogurt or plant-based yogurt

  - Mixed berries (blueberries, strawberries, raspberries)

  - Granola or crushed nuts/seeds

  - Drizzle of honey or maple syrup

b. Oatmeal Power Bowl:

  - Rolled oats cooked with almond milk or water

  - Sliced bananas or other fruit

  - Chia seeds, flaxseeds, and chopped nuts

  - Cinnamon and a drizzle of almond butter

2. Lunch Options

a. Salmon Salad:

  - Grilled salmon on a bed of mixed greens

  - Cherry tomatoes, cucumber, and bell peppers

- Avocado slices and pumpkin seeds

- Lemon vinaigrette dressing

b. Quinoa and Veggie Bowl:

- Cooked quinoa as the base

- Roasted or steamed vegetables (broccoli, carrots, zucchini)

- Chickpeas or black beans for protein

- Tahini or yogurt-based dressing

3.   Dinner Options

a. Stir-Fry Delight:

- Tofu or lean chicken strips stir-fried with colorful vegetables

- Brown rice or whole wheat noodles

- Sesame oil, soy sauce, and ginger for flavor

- Sprinkle of sesame seeds

b. Grilled Veggie Plate:

- Grilled or roasted mixed vegetables (eggplant, peppers, asparagus)

- Quinoa or couscous as the base

- Feta cheese or goat cheese crumbles

- Balsamic vinaigrette dressing

4.   Snack Options

a. Homemade Trail Mix:

- Nuts (almonds, walnuts, cashews)

- Dried fruits (raisins, apricots, cranberries)

- Dark chocolate chips or cacao nibs

- Pumpkin seeds for added crunch

b. Veggie Sticks with Hummus:

- Carrot, cucumber, and bell pepper sticks

- Hummus for dipping

- Optional: Whole grain crackers or whole wheat pita

•Hydration and Lifestyle Considerations

1. Stay Hydrated:

- Drink plenty of water throughout the day to support digestion, skin health, and overall hydration.

2. Limit Added Sugars:

- Minimize the consumption of sugary beverages, desserts, and processed foods.

3. Moderate Caffeine and Alcohol:

- Limit caffeine and alcohol intake to promote better sleep and hormonal balance.

4. Regular Physical Activity:

- Incorporate regular exercise into your routine to support metabolism, bone health, and mood.

Nutrition plays a vital role in promoting well-being and managing the symptoms associated with menopause. By focusing on nutrient-rich foods that provide essential vitamins, minerals, and antioxidants, women can navigate this transformative phase with vitality and resilience. Incorporating calcium-rich foods, omega-3 fatty acids, fiber, and phytoestrogens supports bone health, heart health, and hormonal balance. Nutrient-rich meals such as yogurt parfaits, quinoa bowls, and grilled veggie plates provide both nourishment and pleasure. Combined with hydration and a balanced lifestyle, these dietary choices contribute to a smoother menopausal journey, fostering overall health and a sense of empowerment. By prioritizing proper nutrition

and embracing a wholesome approach to eating, women can thrive during menopause and embrace this transformative phase with strength, energy, and well-being.

Herbal Teas and Infusions

Herbal teas and infusions have been cherished for centuries as natural remedies that offer comfort, relaxation, and a range of health benefits. During the menopausal journey, when hormonal changes and physical transitions occur, incorporating herbal teas into your routine can provide a soothing and holistic approach to managing symptoms and promoting well-being. In this article, we'll explore the benefits of herbal teas for menopause, delve into specific herbs known for their supportive properties, and provide insights on how to create a nourishing herbal tea regimen that enhances your overall health during this transformative phase.

•The Healing Power of Herbal Teas

Herbal teas, also known as tisanes, are brewed by steeping various parts of plants, such as leaves, flowers, roots, and seeds, in hot water. These teas are renowned for their therapeutic properties, which range from calming the mind to aiding digestion and promoting hormonal balance. Incorporating herbal teas into your daily routine can offer a gentle and natural way to address the changes that accompany menopause.

•Benefits of Herbal Teas for Menopause

1. Hormonal Balance
   - Some herbs contain phytoestrogens, which are plant compounds that mimic the effects of estrogen in the body. These compounds can help balance hormone levels during menopause.
2. Mood Support
   - Certain herbs have calming and mood-enhancing properties that can help manage mood swings and promote emotional well-being.
3. Sleep Enhancement
   - Herbal teas can contribute to better sleep quality by calming the nervous system and promoting relaxation.

4. Digestive Comfort
   - Some herbs aid digestion, alleviate bloating, and support overall gut health.

5. Hot Flash Relief
    - Certain herbs with cooling properties can help manage hot flashes and night
      sweats.
6. Bone Health Support
    - Certain herbs are rich in minerals that support bone health and prevent bone loss.

•Notable Herbs for Menopause Wellness

1. Black Cohosh (Cimicifuga racemosa)
    - Known for its potential to reduce hot flashes and improve mood during
      menopause.
2. Red Clover (Trifolium pratense)
    - Contains phytoestrogens that may alleviate hot flashes and promote hormonal
      balance.
3. Sage (Salvia officinalis)
    - Known for its cooling properties and potential to reduce hot flashes and night
      sweats.
4. Chasteberry (Vitex agnus-castus)
    - May help balance hormones and alleviate symptoms such as mood swings and
      irregular periods.
5. Valerian (Valeriana officinalis)
    - Supports relaxation and sleep, making it beneficial for managing insomnia and
      restlessness.
6. Lemon Balm (Melissa officinalis)
    - Offers calming properties that can help reduce stress and anxiety.

•Creating a Nourishing Herbal Tea Regimen

1. Consultation with a Healthcare Professional
    - Before incorporating herbal teas into your routine, consult with a healthcare
      provider, especially if you have any existing health conditions or are taking
      medications.
2. Selecting High-Quality Herbs
    - Choose organic and sustainably sourced herbs to ensure their potency and purity.
3. Single Herbs or Blends
    - Consider whether you want to brew single-herb teas or create custom blends by
      combining herbs with complementary benefits.
4. Brewing Method
    - For most herbal teas, use 1 to 2 teaspoons of dried herbs per cup of hot water.

-    Steep the herbs for about 5 to 10 minutes to extract their beneficial compounds.
5. Adding Flavor
     -    Enhance the flavor of herbal teas with a touch of honey, lemon, or other natural sweeteners.
6. Incorporate Variety
     -    Rotate the herbs you use to benefit from a range of supportive properties.
7. Consistency and Patience
     -    Herbal teas work gradually and may require consistent consumption to notice their effects. Be patient and allow time for the herbs to have an impact.

•Sample Herbal Tea Recipes

1. Calming Lavender Chamomile Tea:

- Ingredients:

  - 1 teaspoon dried lavender flowers

  - 1 teaspoon dried chamomile flowers

- Instructions:

  - Combine the lavender and chamomile in a tea infuser or tea bag.

  - Pour hot water over the herbs and steep for 5 to 10 minutes.

  - Remove the infuser or tea bag and enjoy.

2. Cooling Sage and Peppermint Infusion:

- Ingredients:

  - 1 teaspoon dried sage leaves

  - 1 teaspoon dried peppermint leaves

- Instructions:

  - Mix the sage and peppermint leaves in a tea infuser or tea bag.

  - Pour hot water over the herbs and steep for 5 to 10 minutes.

  - Remove the infuser or tea bag and savor the refreshing infusion.

3. Hormone-Balancing Red Clover Tea:

- Ingredients:

  - 1 tablespoon dried red clover blossoms

  - 1 teaspoon dried nettle leaves

- Instructions:

  - Combine the red clover blossoms and nettle leaves in a tea infuser or tea bag.

  - Pour hot water over the herbs and steep for 10 minutes.

  - Remove the infuser or tea bag and enjoy the nourishing tea.

Herbal teas and infusions offer a gentle and holistic approach to managing the changes that come with menopause. By incorporating herbs with supportive properties into your daily routine, you can promote hormonal balance, enhance mood, and alleviate symptoms like hot flashes and sleep disturbances. Creating a nourishing herbal tea regimen requires careful selection of high-quality herbs, mindful brewing, and a willingness to explore various blends. Remember to consult a healthcare provider before introducing new herbs into your routine, especially if you have underlying health conditions. Embrace the soothing power of herbal teas as a way to support your well-being during this transformative phase of life. With each comforting sip, you can nourish your body, calm your mind, and embrace the journey of menopause with grace and vitality.

Healthy Snacks for Menopause

During this transformative phase, it's essential to nourish your body with nutrient-rich foods that support your well-being. Healthy snacks play a crucial role in maintaining stable energy levels, managing weight, and alleviating symptoms associated with menopause. In this article, we'll explore the importance of healthy snacks during menopause, delve into key nutrients to focus on, and provide practical, delicious snack ideas that cater to your nutritional needs during this journey.

•The Role of Healthy Snacks in Menopause

Maintaining stable blood sugar levels and nourishing your body with balanced nutrients are vital components of managing the symptoms of menopause. Healthy snacks provide a steady source of energy, help prevent overeating during meals, and support overall well-being by addressing specific nutritional requirements during this life stage.

•Key Nutrients to Focus On

1. Fiber
   - Promotes digestive health, prevents constipation, and supports weight management.
2. Protein
   - Aids in muscle maintenance, provides a feeling of fullness, and supports metabolism.
3. Healthy Fats
   - Support hormone production, brain health, and heart health.
4. Calcium and Vitamin D
   - Essential for bone health and prevention of osteoporosis.
5. Antioxidants (Vitamins A, C, E)
   - Protect cells from oxidative stress and support overall health.

•Healthy Snack Ideas

1. Greek Yogurt Parfait:

- Ingredients:

  - Greek yogurt (or plant-based yogurt)

  - Mixed berries (blueberries, strawberries, raspberries)

  - Chia seeds or flaxseeds

  - Chopped nuts (almonds, walnuts)

- Instructions:

  - Layer yogurt, berries, chia seeds, and chopped nuts in a glass or bowl.

  - Drizzle with a touch of honey or maple syrup for added sweetness.

2. Nut Butter and Apple Slices:

- Ingredients:

  - Apple slices

  - Nut butter (almond butter, peanut butter)

- Instructions:

  - Spread nut butter on apple slices for a satisfying combination of protein, fiber, and healthy fats.

3. Hummus and Veggie Sticks:

- Ingredients:

  - Carrot sticks, cucumber slices, bell pepper strips

  - Hummus (classic or flavored)

- Instructions:

  - Dip the veggie sticks in hummus for a crunchy, fiber-rich snack.

4. Trail Mix with a Twist:

- Ingredients:

  - Mixed nuts (almonds, cashews, walnuts)

  - Dried fruits (raisins, apricots, cranberries)

  - Dark chocolate chips or cacao nibs

- Instructions:

  - Combine the nuts, dried fruits, and chocolate in a bowl to create a satisfying and portable snack.

5. Avocado Toast:

- Ingredients:

  - Whole grain toast

  - Avocado slices

  - Sprinkle of sea salt and black pepper

- Instructions:

  - Mash avocado onto the toast and season with salt and pepper for a dose of healthy fats and fiber.

•Hydration and Mindful Snacking

1. Stay Hydrated:
    - Hydrate your body with water throughout the day to support digestion and overall well-being.
2. Mindful Snacking:
    - Pay attention to hunger cues and practice mindful eating to prevent overindulging.
3. Portion Control:
    - Choose portion-controlled snacks to avoid excessive calorie intake.

•Incorporating Hormone-Supportive Ingredients

1. Flaxseeds:
    - Rich in omega-3 fatty acids and lignans that support hormonal balance.
2. Soy Foods:
    - Contain phytoestrogens that can help alleviate menopausal symptoms.

3. Nuts and Seeds:
    - Provide healthy fats and nutrients that support hormone production and overall health.

•Nutrient-Dense Indulgences

1. Dark Chocolate:
    -   Enjoy a small piece of dark chocolate for its antioxidants and mood-boosting properties.

2. Berries:
    -   Snack on berries for their fiber, antioxidants, and natural sweetness.

Healthy snacks are an essential component of a well-rounded menopause wellness plan. By focusing on nutrient-rich foods that provide fiber, protein, healthy fats, and essential vitamins and minerals, you can support stable energy levels, manage weight, and alleviate menopausal symptoms. Incorporating hormone-supportive ingredients like flaxseeds and soy foods can provide additional benefits during this transformative phase. Remember to hydrate adequately and practice mindful snacking to maintain a balanced approach to nutrition. Whether you're reaching for a yogurt parfait, enjoying avocado toast, or savoring a handful of mixed nuts, each nourishing bite contributes to your overall well-being and vitality. Embrace the power of healthy snacks as a way to care for your body, enhance your energy levels, and navigate menopause with a sense of empowerment and self-care.

Chapter Nine

Personalizing Your Menopause Journey

Tailoring the Natural Approach to Your Needs

Menopause is a unique and transformative phase in a woman's life that brings about a variety of physical, emotional, and hormonal changes. The natural approach to managing menopause offers a holistic way to navigate these changes and support your well-being. However, every woman's experience of menopause is different, and tailoring the natural approach to your individual needs is essential for optimal results. In this article, we'll explore the importance of personalization in the natural approach to menopause, delve into ways to customize your strategies, and provide insights into how embracing your uniqueness can enhance your menopause journey.

•The Power of Personalization

Personalization is a powerful tool that can greatly benefit women going through menopause. Menopause is a unique experience for each individual, with symptoms ranging from hot flashes and mood swings to sleep disturbances and vaginal dryness. By personalizing their approach to managing menopause, women can find strategies and treatments that work best for them.

One aspect of personalization in menopause is understanding and acknowledging the individual's specific symptoms and needs. What works for one woman may not work for another, so it's important to tailor treatments and lifestyle changes accordingly. This may involve consulting with healthcare professionals who specialize in menopause or seeking alternative therapies such as acupuncture or herbal remedies.

Another aspect of personalization is recognizing that menopause affects more than just physical symptoms. Emotional well-being and mental health can also be impacted during this time. Therefore, it's crucial to address these aspects of menopause as well. This may involve seeking support from friends, family, or support groups, as well as practicing self-care activities that promote relaxation and stress reduction.

Personalization also extends to lifestyle modifications that can help manage menopause symptoms. This may include adjusting diet and exercise routines, as well as incorporating stress management techniques such as meditation or yoga. By tailoring these lifestyle changes to individual preferences and needs, women can optimize their overall well-being during menopause.

Furthermore, personalization in menopause involves staying informed and educated about the latest research and treatment options. By being proactive in seeking information, women can

make informed decisions about their health and choose the most effective strategies for managing their symptoms.

The power of personalization in menopause lies in recognizing that each woman's experience is unique and tailoring treatments, lifestyle changes, and support systems to meet individual needs. By embracing personalization, women can empower themselves to navigate through menopause with greater control and improved quality of life. Remember to consult with healthcare professionals for personalized advice and guidance throughout this journey.

•Identifying Your Unique Needs

1. Self-Assessment:
   - Reflect on your current health, lifestyle, and menopausal symptoms. What are your main concerns and goals?
   - Consider your physical, emotional, and mental well-being as you assess your needs.
2. Health History:
   - Review your medical history and any existing health conditions. Are there specific areas that require extra attention?
   - Consulting with a healthcare provider can provide insights into potential challenges and opportunities for natural management.
3. Lifestyle and Preferences:
   - Take into account your daily routines, dietary preferences, exercise habits, and stress levels.
   - Consider what types of natural approaches align with your lifestyle and resonate with your values.

•Customizing Your Natural Approach

1. Diet and Nutrition:
   - Tailor your diet to address specific concerns. For example, focus on bone-supporting foods if bone health is a priority.

- Incorporate foods rich in nutrients that align with your needs, such as omega-3 fatty acids, phytoestrogens, and antioxidants.

2. Herbal Support:
   - Choose herbs based on your symptoms and preferences. For instance, if hot flashes are an issue, opt for herbs known for their cooling properties.
   - Experiment with different herbal teas and supplements to find what works best for you.

3. Lifestyle Modifications:
   - Customize your exercise routine to include activities that you enjoy and that support your overall health.
   - Incorporate stress-relief practices that resonate with you, whether it's meditation, yoga, or spending time in nature.

4. Mind-Body Connection:
   - Tailor mindfulness and meditation practices to your preferences. Explore various techniques to find what helps you manage stress and enhance self-awareness.
   - Consider integrating practices that promote emotional well-being and self-acceptance.

5. Sleep Strategies:
   - Experiment with sleep hygiene practices to improve your sleep quality. Adjust your bedtime routine and sleep environment to suit your needs.
   - Incorporate relaxation techniques before bed to promote restful sleep.

6. Seeking Professional Guidance:
   - Consult with healthcare providers who understand and support the natural approach to menopause. Collaborate with them to create a personalized plan.
   - Consider working with holistic practitioners, such as naturopaths, acupuncturists, or integrative health coaches.

•Embracing Your Uniqueness

1. Self-Care and Self-Compassion:
   - Embrace self-care practices that nourish your body and soul. Treat yourself with kindness and compassion.
   - Acknowledge that your needs may change over time, and be open to adjusting your approach accordingly.

2. Listening to Your Body:
   - Tune into your body's signals and responses. Pay attention to how different strategies impact your well-being.
   - Trust your intuition and make choices that align with your body's wisdom.

3. Empowerment and Ownership:
    -   Recognize that you are the expert of your own experience. Empower yourself to make informed decisions about your natural approach.
    -   Take ownership of your health and well-being by actively engaging in your journey.

•Celebrate Your Progress

1. Small Wins:
    -   Celebrate each step forward, no matter how small. Your progress is a testament to your dedication and effort.
    -   Keeping a journal can help you track your achievements and milestones.
2. Holistic Growth:
    -   Embrace the holistic growth that comes with tailoring the natural approach to your needs.
    -   As you navigate menopause, you're not just addressing physical changes but also fostering personal growth and self-discovery.

Tailoring the natural approach to menopause to your unique needs is a powerful way to enhance your well-being and navigate this transformative phase with grace and empowerment. By identifying your individual requirements, customizing your strategies, and embracing your uniqueness, you create a path that aligns with your body, mind, and soul. Whether you're adjusting your diet, exploring herbal support, or nurturing the mind-body connection, your personalized approach reflects your commitment to holistic health. As you celebrate your progress and honor your journey, you not only manage menopause naturally but also embark on a transformative experience that nurtures self-discovery, self-compassion, and personal growth. Your customized journey through menopause is a testament to your strength, resilience, and dedication to nurturing your well-being in a way that honors your individuality.

Tracking Progress and Adjustments

As you journey through this transformative phase, tracking your progress and making necessary adjustments become essential components of managing your well-being effectively. By staying attuned to your body, emotions, and overall health, you can navigate menopause with greater awareness and make informed decisions about your natural approach. In this article, we'll delve into the importance of tracking progress and adjustments during menopause, explore key areas to monitor, and provide insights into how this practice can empower you on your journey of self-care and well-being.

•The Value of Tracking Progress

Tracking progress during menopause can be incredibly valuable for several reasons. Menopause is a transitional phase in a woman's life that can bring about various physical and emotional changes. By tracking progress, women can gain insights into their symptoms, monitor the effectiveness of treatments, and make informed decisions about their health and well-being.

One of the primary benefits of tracking progress in menopause is gaining a better understanding of individual symptoms and their patterns. Menopause symptoms can vary greatly from woman to woman and even day to day. By keeping track of symptoms such as hot flashes, mood swings, sleep disturbances, and vaginal dryness, women can identify triggers, patterns, and potential correlations. This information can help them make lifestyle adjustments, seek appropriate treatments, and better manage their symptoms.

Tracking progress can also provide a sense of control and empowerment during the menopause journey. Menopause can be a challenging and unpredictable time, but by actively monitoring and recording symptoms, women can take an active role in their own health. This sense of control can help alleviate anxiety and stress, as well as provide a sense of accomplishment as women see improvements or positive changes over time.

Additionally, tracking progress allows women to assess the effectiveness of treatments and interventions. Menopause management often involves a combination of lifestyle changes, hormone therapy, and alternative therapies. By keeping track of symptoms and treatment approaches, women can evaluate what works best for them and make adjustments as needed. This can save time, money, and potential side effects by avoiding treatments that may not be effective or necessary.

Moreover, tracking progress can be helpful when seeking medical advice or consulting with healthcare professionals. By having a record of symptoms and their frequency, women can provide accurate and detailed information to their healthcare providers. This can facilitate more productive and targeted discussions, leading to personalized treatment plans that address specific needs and concerns.

Tracking progress also allows women to celebrate milestones and achievements. Menopause is a journey, and it's important to acknowledge and celebrate progress along the way. Whether it's a reduction in hot flashes, improved sleep quality, or better overall well-being, tracking progress can provide tangible evidence of positive changes and motivate women to continue their efforts in managing menopause.

Tracking progress in menopause offers numerous benefits. From gaining insights into symptoms and patterns to evaluating treatment effectiveness and empowering women to take an active role in their health, tracking progress is a valuable tool for navigating the menopause journey. It provides a sense of control, helps in making informed decisions, and facilitates effective communication with healthcare professionals. By tracking symptoms, women can better understand their bodies, identify triggers, and make necessary adjustments to improve their overall well-being. So, whether it's through journaling, using mobile apps, or keeping a calendar,

tracking progress can be a powerful tool in managing and embracing the changes that come with menopause.

•Areas to Monitor and Track

1. Physical Symptoms:
   - Record any physical changes you experience, such as hot flashes, night sweats, sleep disturbances, changes in energy levels, and changes in weight.
2. Emotional Well-Being:
   - Document your emotional state and mood fluctuations. Are you experiencing mood swings, irritability, anxiety, or feelings of sadness?
3. Digestive Health:
   - Monitor any changes in digestion, bloating, and discomfort after meals.
4. Sleep Patterns:
   - Track your sleep quality and duration. Are you experiencing insomnia, difficulty falling asleep, or waking up frequently during the night?
5. Hormonal Changes:
   - Note any irregularities in your menstrual cycle if applicable. If you're postmenopausal, observe changes related to hormonal shifts.
6. Nutritional Choices:
   - Keep a food diary to document your dietary choices and identify patterns that may be affecting your well-being.
7. Stress Levels:
   - Monitor your stress levels and sources of stress. How are stress and anxiety impacting your overall health?

9. Exercise Routine:
   - Document your exercise habits and how they impact your energy levels, mood, and physical well-being.
10. Herbal Remedies:
   - If you're incorporating herbal teas or supplements, track how they affect your symptoms and overall health.

•The Benefits of Tracking Progress

1. Informed Decision-Making:
   - Tracking your progress allows you to make informed decisions about adjustments to your natural approach.
   - You can identify strategies that are working well and those that may need modification.

2. Early Detection of Patterns:
   - Documenting changes over time helps you recognize patterns and correlations between different factors.
   - For example, you might notice that certain foods trigger hot flashes or that certain stressors impact your sleep quality.
3. Empowerment and Control:
   - By actively engaging in tracking your progress, you regain a sense of control over your health and well-being.
   - You become an active participant in your journey, rather than a passive observer.
4. Healthcare Collaboration:
   - If you're working with healthcare providers, tracking your progress provides them with valuable information to guide their recommendations.
   - Collaborating with professionals becomes more effective when you can share specific insights about your experiences.

•Making Adjustments with Intention

1. Analyze Your Data:
   - Review your progress notes to identify patterns and trends. Are there specific triggers or factors that consistently impact your well-being?
2. Prioritize Changes:
   - Determine which aspects of your natural approach need adjustment based on the areas that are most affecting your quality of life.

3. Gradual Changes:
    - When making adjustments, consider making gradual changes to assess their impact before fully committing.
4. Consultation with Professionals:
    - If you're uncertain about adjustments or need guidance, consult with healthcare providers who understand the natural approach to menopause.
5. Holistic Approach:
    - Address adjustments holistically, taking into account the mind-body connection, nutrition, exercise, stress management, and emotional well-being.

•Empowering Your Journey

1. Celebrate Progress:
    - Acknowledge and celebrate the positive changes and improvements you observe along your menopause journey.
    - Celebrating progress enhances motivation and positivity.

2. Embrace Flexibility:
    - Recognize that adjustments are a natural part of any journey. Embrace the flexibility to adapt as needed.
3. Self-Compassion:
    - Approach adjustments with self-compassion and an understanding that your well-being is a priority.
4. Mindfulness and Self-Awareness:
    - Cultivate mindfulness and self-awareness as you navigate changes and make adjustments.
    - Tuning into your body's responses and honoring your needs enhance your ability to make effective decisions.

Tracking progress and making adjustments during menopause is an empowering practice that allows you to navigate this transformative phase with greater awareness and intention. By monitoring various aspects of your health, observing patterns, and collaborating with healthcare professionals when needed, you can fine-tune your natural approach to match your unique needs. Adjustments are not setbacks but rather opportunities for growth, self-discovery, and enhanced well-being. Embrace the journey with openness and flexibility, celebrating your progress and making choices that honor your body, mind, and spirit. As you track your progress and make informed adjustments, you embark on a journey of empowerment, resilience, and self-care that will serve you well during and beyond menopause.

Chapter Ten

Looking Ahead

Post-Menopausal Health Considerations

Post-menopause marks the phase of a woman's life after she has completed the transition through menopause, a period characterized by the cessation of menstruation and significant hormonal changes. While menopause itself is a transformative journey, post-menopause brings about a new set of health considerations. During this stage, women continue to experience changes in their bodies and well-being, and focusing on holistic health becomes essential to thriving in this next chapter of life. In this article, we'll delve into key post-menopausal health considerations, explore strategies for maintaining well-being, and provide insights into how embracing this phase can lead to a fulfilling and vibrant post-menopausal journey.

•Embracing Post-Menopause

Post-menopause is not an endpoint but rather a new beginning. It's a time to embrace the wisdom, experiences, and opportunities that come with this phase. While there are certain health changes to be aware of, post-menopause can also be a period of empowerment, self-discovery, and the pursuit of passions that may have taken a backseat during earlier life stages.

•Understanding Post-Menopausal Health Considerations

1. Bone Health:
   - After menopause, the risk of osteoporosis increases due to decreased estrogen levels.
   - Focus on maintaining bone health through calcium-rich foods, vitamin D, weight-bearing exercises, and regular bone density screenings.
2. Heart Health:
   - Cardiovascular disease risk rises post-menopause.
   - Adopt heart-healthy habits, such as maintaining a balanced diet, engaging in regular physical activity, managing stress, and avoiding smoking.
3. Weight Management:
   - Metabolism often slows down post-menopause, which can lead to weight gain.
   - Prioritize a balanced diet, portion control, and regular physical activity to support weight management.
4. Hormonal Changes:
   - Hormone levels continue to fluctuate post-menopause, affecting mood, energy levels, and overall well-being.

   - Focus on stress management, regular exercise, and a balanced diet to support hormonal balance.
5. Vaginal Health:
   - Vaginal dryness and thinning of vaginal tissues can occur post-menopause due to declining estrogen levels.
   - Use water-based lubricants, consider vaginal moisturizers, and speak to a healthcare provider about potential treatments.
6. Mental and Emotional Health:
   - Mood swings, anxiety, and depression can persist post-menopause.
   - Prioritize self-care, engage in stress-relief activities, maintain social connections, and consider professional support if needed.
7. Cognitive Health:
   - Post-menopausal women may experience changes in memory and cognitive function.
   - Stay mentally active through puzzles, reading, learning new skills, and maintaining a healthy lifestyle.

•Strategies for Post-Menopausal Well-Being

1. Nutrition and Hydration:
   - Focus on a balanced diet rich in nutrient-dense foods, including whole grains, lean proteins, fruits, vegetables, and healthy fats.
   - Stay hydrated to support overall health and organ function.
2. Physical Activity:
   - Engage in regular exercise to support bone health, cardiovascular fitness, weight management, and overall well-being.
   - Include a mix of cardiovascular exercises, strength training, and flexibility activities.
3. Stress Management:
   - Practice stress-relief techniques such as meditation, deep breathing, yoga, and mindfulness to support emotional well-being.
4. Social Connections:
   - Maintain social interactions to promote mental and emotional health.
   - Stay connected with friends, family, and engage in social activities.
5. Regular Check-Ups:
   - Continue to schedule regular check-ups and screenings to monitor your health, including bone density tests, cholesterol checks, and mammograms.
6. Sleep Hygiene:
   - Prioritize sleep hygiene practices to support restful sleep and overall well-being.
   - Create a calming bedtime routine, limit screen time before bed, and create a comfortable sleep environment.

7. Mind-Body Practices:
   - Engage in practices that nurture the mind-body connection, such as yoga, meditation, tai chi, and qigong.

•Embracing Fulfillment in Post-Menopause

1. Pursue Passions:
   - Use post-menopause as an opportunity to explore interests and passions that may have been sidelined during other life stages.
2. Lifelong Learning:
   - Engage in lifelong learning to stimulate cognitive function and expand your horizons.
3. Volunteering and Community Involvement:
   - Get involved in your community through volunteering or participating in local events.
4. Embracing Change:

- Embrace the physical and emotional changes of post-menopause as part of a natural progression.
        - Celebrate the wisdom and insights gained from your experiences.
5. Maintaining Relationships:
        - Nurture relationships with loved ones and seek new connections that align with your post-menopausal journey.

Post-menopause is a chapter of life that presents both health considerations and opportunities for growth. By understanding the changes that may occur in areas such as bone health, heart health, and emotional well-being, you can take proactive steps to support your overall well-being. Adopting healthy lifestyle habits, engaging in physical activity, managing stress, and maintaining regular check-ups contribute to a vibrant post-menopausal life. Embrace the unique qualities of this phase, such as newfound freedom, wisdom, and the ability to pursue passions with renewed vigor. Thriving beyond menopause is not only achievable but also a testament to your resilience, self-care, and commitment to embracing the journey of life in all its stages. With a holistic approach to well-being, you can navigate post-menopause with grace, empowerment, and a deep sense of fulfillment.

Continuation of Healthy Habits

As you navigate through this significant transition, maintaining healthy habits becomes even more crucial to support your overall well-being. The continuation of healthy practices during menopause is not only beneficial for managing symptoms but also for promoting long-term health and vitality. In this article, we'll explore the importance of sustaining healthy habits during menopause, provide insights into specific areas of focus, and offer strategies to help you thrive through this life stage.

•The Menopause Journey: A Time for Self-Care

Menopause is a unique journey, and it presents an opportunity to prioritize self-care and wellness. By continuing healthy habits that align with your body's changing needs, you can navigate this phase with grace, empowerment, and a sense of control over your well-being. The positive impact of these practices can extend far beyond menopause, contributing to a vibrant and fulfilling life.

•The Importance of Continuation

1. Symptom Management:
   - Sustaining healthy habits can help alleviate common menopausal symptoms such as hot flashes, mood swings, sleep disturbances, and weight changes.
2. Long-Term Health Benefits:
   - Healthy habits established during menopause can contribute to preventing chronic conditions like heart disease, osteoporosis, and diabetes later in life.
3. Physical Resilience:
   - Continuing physical activity and a balanced diet can support your body's resilience, maintain muscle mass, bone density, and joint health.
4. Mental and Emotional Well-Being:
   - Healthy habits play a pivotal role in managing stress, anxiety, and mood swings often associated with menopause.
5. Quality of Life:
   - Sustaining well-being practices enhances your quality of life, helping you remain active, engaged, and emotionally fulfilled.

•Areas of Focus and Strategies

1. Physical Activity:
   - Focus: Regular exercise supports bone health, cardiovascular fitness, weight management, and overall vitality.
   - Strategies: Engage in a mix of aerobic exercises, strength training, and flexibility activities. Choose activities you enjoy to ensure consistency.
2. Nutrition:
   - Focus: A balanced diet rich in nutrients supports hormonal balance, bone health, and energy levels.
   - Strategies: Prioritize whole foods such as fruits, vegetables, lean proteins, whole grains, and healthy fats. Stay hydrated and listen to your body's hunger cues.
3. Stress Management:

- Focus: Managing stress is essential for emotional well-being and hormonal balance.
  - Strategies: Practice relaxation techniques such as meditation, deep breathing, and mindfulness. Engage in activities you find calming and enjoyable.
4. Sleep Quality:
   - Focus: Quality sleep is crucial for overall health and symptom management.
   - Strategies: Maintain a consistent sleep schedule, create a relaxing bedtime routine, and ensure your sleep environment is comfortable.
5. Mind-Body Connection:
   - Focus: Cultivating the mind-body connection supports emotional equilibrium and overall wellness.
   - Strategies: Engage in practices like yoga, tai chi, and meditation. These activities enhance self-awareness and stress relief.
6. Social Connections:
   - Focus: Nurturing social connections fosters emotional support and a sense of belonging.
   - Strategies: Stay connected with friends, family, and engage in social activities that bring you joy and fulfillment.

•Navigating Hormonal Changes

1. Hormone-Balancing Foods:
   - Focus: Certain foods can support hormonal balance during menopause.
   - Strategies: Incorporate foods rich in phytoestrogens, omega-3 fatty acids, and antioxidants. Examples include flaxseeds, soy, fatty fish, and colorful fruits and vegetables.

2. Herbal Support:
   - Focus: Herbal remedies can aid in managing menopausal symptoms and promoting well-being.
   - Strategies: Consult with a healthcare provider before using herbal supplements. Some commonly used herbs include black cohosh, dong quai, and red clover.

•Maintaining Bone and Heart Health

1. Bone Health:

- Focus: Postmenopausal women are at higher risk of osteoporosis. Prioritize bone health to prevent fractures and maintain mobility.
   - Strategies: Consume calcium-rich foods, engage in weight-bearing exercises, and consider vitamin D supplementation if necessary.
2. Heart Health:
   - Focus: Cardiovascular risks can increase during menopause due to hormonal changes.
   - Strategies: Maintain a heart-healthy diet by reducing saturated fats and sodium. Engage in regular aerobic exercise and monitor blood pressure and cholesterol levels.

•Professional Guidance and Self-Care

1. Regular Check-Ups:
   - Focus: Regular medical check-ups are essential for monitoring health and addressing concerns.
   - Strategies: Schedule regular appointments with healthcare providers to assess your well-being and discuss any changes or challenges.
2. Hormone Replacement Therapy (HRT):
   - Focus: Hormone replacement therapy may be considered to manage severe menopausal symptoms.
   - Strategies: Consult with a healthcare provider to determine if HRT is appropriate for your situation, considering the potential risks and benefits.

•Embracing Holistic Well-Being

1. Mindful Aging:
   - Focus: Embrace the aging process with a positive mindset and self-compassion.
   - Strategies: Celebrate your wisdom and life experiences. Focus on personal growth, lifelong learning, and finding joy in the present moment.
2. Self-Care Rituals:
   - Focus: Self-care rituals enhance emotional well-being and self-nurturing.

- Strategies: Engage in activities that bring you joy, whether it's reading, taking long baths, or indulging in hobbies.

Continuing healthy habits during menopause is a testament to your commitment to self-care and overall well-being. By focusing on physical activity, nutrition, stress management, and emotional equilibrium, you empower yourself to navigate this transformative phase with grace and vitality. As you maintain a holistic approach to wellness, you create a foundation for a fulfilling and vibrant life beyond menopause. The journey through menopause is not merely about managing symptoms but about embracing your strength, wisdom, and capacity for growth. By sustaining healthy habits, you embark on a lifelong adventure of self-discovery, empowerment, and well-being that transcends age and stages.

Inspiring Others on the Menopausal Journey

As you navigate through this unique transition, you have the power to inspire and uplift others who are on a similar path. Sharing your experiences, insights, and strategies can create a supportive community that empowers women to embrace their individual journeys with grace and confidence. In this article, we'll explore the significance of inspiring others during the menopausal journey, offer insights into effective ways to provide support, and discuss how your guidance can foster a sense of camaraderie and empowerment.

•The Power of Shared Experiences

The menopausal journey is personal yet universal, as countless women across different cultures and backgrounds undergo similar changes. By sharing your experiences and lessons learned, you create a space where others can feel understood, validated, and less alone in their challenges.

Your journey becomes a source of inspiration that encourages others to embrace their uniqueness and navigate menopause with a sense of community.

•The Importance of Inspiring Others

1. Reducing Stigma:
   - Sharing your experiences helps break down the stigma surrounding menopause and encourages open conversations about this natural phase of life.
2. Validation and Empathy:
   - By sharing your challenges and triumphs, you validate the experiences of others, fostering empathy and creating a safe space for discussion.
3. Promoting Self-Care:
   - Inspiring others to prioritize self-care during menopause emphasizes the importance of holistic well-being and empowers them to prioritize their health.
4. Fostering Connection:
   - Building a community of women who support and uplift one another creates a sense of connection and camaraderie.

•Ways to Inspire and Support

1. Open and Honest Conversations:
   - Engage in open discussions about menopause with friends, family, and acquaintances. By sharing your own experiences, you invite others to share theirs.
2. Online Platforms:
   - Utilize social media, blogs, or online forums to share your journey, insights, and advice. Your words can reach a broader audience and provide valuable support.
3. Organize Support Groups:
   - Create or join local menopause support groups where women can come together to share experiences, exchange advice, and provide emotional support.
4. Workshops and Seminars:
   - Host workshops or seminars on menopause-related topics to educate and empower women with information and practical strategies.
5. Writing and Publications:
   - Write articles, essays, or even a book detailing your menopausal journey and the lessons you've learned. Your words can offer guidance and comfort to others.

•Sharing Personal Insights

1. Challenges and Triumphs:

- Share your personal challenges during menopause and how you overcame them. Highlight moments of triumph and personal growth.
2. Mind-Body Connection:
   - Discuss how practices like mindfulness, meditation, and yoga have supported your emotional well-being and stress management.
3. Nutrition and Lifestyle:
   - Offer insights into how your dietary choices and lifestyle adjustments have positively impacted your menopausal experience.
4. Self-Care Strategies:
   - Share self-care rituals that have helped you navigate menopause with grace, whether it's journaling, spending time in nature, or engaging in hobbies.
5. Relationships and Communication:
   - Discuss how you've navigated changes in relationships and communication during menopause, offering guidance on effective ways to communicate your needs.

•Empowering Others Through Positive Change

1. Celebrating Diversity:
   - Embrace and celebrate the diversity of menopausal experiences. Encourage women to share their unique journeys without judgment.
2. Fostering Self-Compassion:
   - Inspire self-compassion by sharing how you've learned to be kind to yourself during moments of difficulty or self-doubt.
3. Encouraging Self-Discovery:
   - Emphasize the opportunity for self-discovery during menopause and encourage others to explore new passions, interests, and hobbies.
4. Promoting Body Positivity:
   - Advocate for body positivity by highlighting the beauty and strength that come with age and embracing the changes that menopause brings.

•Supporting Men in Understanding Menopause

1. Educating Partners and Loved Ones:
   - Share information about menopause with your partners, family members, and friends. Encourage empathy and understanding.

2. Inviting Dialogue:

- Initiate open conversations with the men in your life about menopause. Invite them to ask questions and learn alongside you.

As you navigate the menopausal journey, you have the opportunity to inspire and uplift others through your experiences and insights. By sharing openly and honestly, you create a supportive community that reduces stigma, promotes well-being, and empowers women to embrace their unique paths. Through conversations, online platforms, workshops, and writing, you can offer guidance on navigating challenges, fostering resilience, and prioritizing self-care. By fostering connection, validating experiences, and promoting positivity, you contribute to a movement of empowerment that transcends age and background. Your willingness to share your journey inspires others to embrace their own transformations with grace, confidence, and a sense of camaraderie.

Chapter Eleven

Resources

Recommended Reading

Menopause is a transformative phase that presents both challenges and opportunities for growth and empowerment. As you embark on this journey, seeking knowledge and understanding can greatly enhance your experience and well-being. Fortunately, there is a wealth of literature available that offers insights, guidance, and practical advice for navigating menopause with grace and confidence. In this article, we'll explore a curated list of recommended reading resources that cover a wide range of topics related to menopause, from hormonal changes to emotional well-being, nutrition, and holistic health. These resources will empower you to approach menopause as a time of growth, self-discovery, and vibrant well-being.

1. "The Wisdom of Menopause" by Christiane Northrup, M.D.

    - In this comprehensive guide, Dr. Christiane Northrup provides a holistic perspective on menopause. She addresses physical, emotional, and spiritual aspects of this phase while offering empowering insights for embracing the changes with wisdom and vitality.

2. "Menopause Confidential" by Tara Allmen, M.D.

    - Dr. Tara Allmen, a leading expert in menopause, offers practical advice and evidence-based information in a conversational style. The book covers a range of topics, from hormone therapy to sexuality, providing a clear and accessible resource for women navigating menopause.

3. "The Menopause Manifesto" by Dr. Jen Gunter

    - Dr. Jen Gunter, an outspoken advocate for women's health, delves into the scientific and cultural aspects of menopause. With a mix of science and humor, she addresses common myths and provides a guide to understanding and managing menopausal changes.

4. Goddesses Never Age" by Christiane Northrup, M.D.

    - While not solely focused on menopause, this book by Dr. Christiane Northrup explores the concept of aging with vitality, embracing the wisdom and beauty that come with each life stage. It offers insights into how to live a fulfilling and empowered life as you age.

5. "The Hormone Fix" by Anna Cabeca, D.O.

- Dr. Anna Cabeca offers a comprehensive guide to addressing hormonal imbalances during menopause. Through dietary recommendations, lifestyle changes, and natural therapies, she empowers women to take control of their hormone health and overall well-being.

6. "Menopause: A Natural and Spiritual Journey" by Rosetta Reitz

- This book offers a holistic perspective on menopause, emphasizing its spiritual and emotional dimensions. Rosetta Reitz guides women through the emotional shifts of menopause and explores the potential for personal growth and transformation.

7. "The Hot Flash Club" series by Nancy Thayer

- For a lighthearted and fictional take on menopause, the "Hot Flash Club" series follows a group of women as they navigate the challenges and joys of midlife. The series offers humor, camaraderie, and relatable experiences.

8. "Menopause Confidential: A Doctor Reveals the Secrets to Thriving Through Midlife" by Dr. Jennifer Ashton

- Written by Dr. Jennifer Ashton, a board-certified OB-GYN, this book provides a comprehensive and empowering guide to navigating menopause. It covers a wide range of topics, including hormonal changes, symptoms, and practical strategies for thriving during this life stage.

9. "The Menopause Book: The Complete Guide: Hormones, Hot Flashes, Health, Moods, Sleep, Sex" by Barbara Kantrowitz and Pat Wingert

- This comprehensive guide covers various aspects of menopause, including hormonal changes, physical symptoms, mental health, and sexual well-being. It offers evidence-based information and practical advice for women seeking to understand and manage menopause.

10. "The Harvard Guide to Women's Health" by Karen J. Carlson, Stephanie A. Eisenstat, and Terra Zipory.

- Although not exclusively focused on menopause, this guide provides valuable information on women's health at all stages of life, including menopause. It covers a wide range of topics, from medical advice to self-care practices and emotional well-being.

These recommended reading resources offer a diverse range of perspectives and insights into navigating menopause with empowerment, wisdom, and well-being. Whether you're seeking practical advice, scientific understanding, emotional support, or even a touch of humor, these books provide valuable guidance for embracing the menopausal journey. As you explore these resources, you'll find yourself equipped with knowledge, inspiration, and a sense of community

as you navigate the changes and opportunities that menopause brings. Remember that every woman's journey is unique, and these resources can serve as companions and guides as you embark on this transformative phase with confidence and grace.

Websites and Online Communities

In the digital age, seeking support, information, and community has never been easier, especially for women navigating the complexities of menopause. Online platforms provide a wealth of resources, advice, and connections to empower women during this transformative phase. From informative websites to vibrant online communities, the virtual world offers a space where women can find understanding, share experiences, and gain valuable insights. In this article, we'll explore a selection of websites and online communities that cater to menopausal women, offering a range of resources for empowerment, well-being, and camaraderie.

1. Menopause.org

   - Run by The North American Menopause Society (NAMS), Menopause.org is a trusted source of evidence-based information on menopause and its various aspects. The website provides articles, videos, and resources covering hormonal changes, symptoms, treatments, and overall wellness. It's an ideal starting point for women seeking accurate and up-to-date information.

2. Women's Health Concern – Menopause

   - Women's Health Concern offers a dedicated section on menopause, providing comprehensive information on the stages of menopause, hormonal changes, symptom management, and lifestyle advice. The website includes downloadable resources and a helpline for women seeking personalized guidance.

3. Healthline – Menopause

   - Healthline's menopause section offers a range of articles written by medical professionals and experts. It covers topics such as symptoms, treatments, and self-care practices. The website also includes personal stories and experiences shared by women who have gone through menopause.

4. MyMenopauseCommunity

- MyMenopauseCommunity is an online platform where women can connect with others going through similar experiences. The platform offers discussion forums, blogs, and expert articles on various menopause-related topics. It's a space to share stories, ask questions, and provide support to one another.

5. Menopause Matters Forum

- The Menopause Matters Forum is an active online community where women can engage in discussions about menopause and related health issues. It's a supportive environment where women can ask questions, share experiences, and receive advice from others who have been through similar situations.

6. The Silvers

- The Silvers is an online community that focuses on embracing the wisdom and beauty that come with age, including menopause. It features articles, interviews, and stories that celebrate the vibrant lives of women over 50. The platform encourages self-expression, positivity, and empowerment.

7. MenoPause Blog

- MenoPause Blog is a space where women can find a wide range of articles covering menopause-related topics. From nutrition and exercise to mental health and lifestyle adjustments, the blog offers practical advice and insights to help women navigate the menopausal journey.

8. Red Hot Mamas

- Red Hot Mamas offers a blend of educational resources and community engagement. The website provides information on menopause, along with health quizzes, webinars, and a "Chat with the Experts" feature. It's a supportive platform for women seeking to enhance their knowledge and well-being during menopause.

9. HealthUnlocked – Menopause Matters

- HealthUnlocked hosts a Menopause Matters community where women can connect, share stories, and ask questions in a safe and supportive space. Members can seek advice from others who have experienced menopause and engage in discussions on various topics.

10. The Menopause Exchange

- The Menopause Exchange offers evidence-based information and resources on menopause. The website includes articles, newsletters, and a "Your Stories" section where women can share their personal experiences and insights about navigating menopause.

Websites and online communities for menopause offer a valuable virtual space where women can access information, share experiences, and connect with others who are on a similar journey. From educational resources to supportive communities, these online platforms empower women to embrace menopause with knowledge, confidence, and a sense of camaraderie. Whether you're seeking advice on symptom management, lifestyle adjustments, or emotional well-being, these websites and communities provide a wealth of insights and connections that can enhance your menopausal experience. Remember that every woman's journey is unique, and the online world offers a multitude of resources to help you navigate this transformative phase with grace and empowerment.

Professional Services and Practitioners

Navigating menopause involves not only personal adjustments but also seeking guidance from qualified professionals who specialize in women's health and well-being during this transformative phase. From medical practitioners to alternative therapists, a range of professionals offer their expertise to help women manage symptoms, make informed decisions, and promote holistic health. In this article, we'll explore the various professional services and practitioners available to support women during menopause, highlighting their roles and contributions to enhancing women's overall well-being.

1. Gynecologists and Obstetricians:

- Gynecologists and obstetricians are medical doctors who specialize in women's reproductive health. They play a crucial role in guiding women through menopause, offering medical assessments, discussing hormonal therapy options, and addressing any health concerns that may arise during this phase.

2. Menopause Specialists:

- Menopause specialists are healthcare professionals who have specialized training and expertise in menopause-related issues. They provide comprehensive care, offer personalized treatment plans, and help women navigate the physical and emotional changes associated with menopause.

3. Endocrinologists:

- Endocrinologists are medical doctors who specialize in hormones and the endocrine system. They can assess hormonal imbalances, provide guidance on

  hormone replacement therapy, and address conditions such as thyroid disorders that may affect menopause.

4. Integrative Medicine Practitioners:

- Integrative medicine practitioners combine conventional medical practices with alternative and complementary therapies. They offer a holistic approach to managing menopause symptoms by considering factors such as nutrition, stress management, and mind-body practices.

5. Nutritionists and Dietitians:

- Nutritionists and dietitians can help women create tailored dietary plans to manage menopause-related changes and promote overall health. They offer insights into nutrient-rich foods, hydration, and dietary strategies to support hormonal balance.

6. Mental Health Professionals:

- Psychologists, therapists, and counselors specialize in mental health and can provide essential support for managing the emotional aspects of menopause. They offer coping strategies, stress management techniques, and a safe space to discuss feelings and concerns.

7. Acupuncturists:

- Acupuncturists use traditional Chinese medicine techniques to stimulate specific points on the body. Acupuncture can help alleviate menopause symptoms such as hot flashes, sleep disturbances, and mood swings.

8. Naturopathic Doctors:

- Naturopathic doctors focus on natural and holistic approaches to health. They can provide guidance on herbal remedies, supplements, and lifestyle adjustments to manage menopause symptoms.

9. Physical Therapists:

- Physical therapists specialize in improving mobility and addressing musculoskeletal issues. For women experiencing changes in bone density or joint health during menopause, physical therapists can provide exercises and strategies to maintain physical well-being.

10. Sex Therapists:

- Sex therapists specialize in addressing sexual concerns and intimacy issues. They can help women navigate changes in libido, vaginal dryness, and other sexual health concerns that may arise during menopause.

11. Fitness and Yoga Instructors:

- Fitness trainers and yoga instructors who specialize in women's health can guide women through appropriate exercises that support bone health, flexibility, and overall fitness during menopause.

12. Support Groups and Menopause Coaches:

- Support groups and menopause coaches provide a sense of community and guidance through peer interactions. Coaches offer personalized advice and strategies to navigate menopause with empowerment.

Professional services and practitioners play a vital role in guiding women through the menopausal journey. These experts offer medical assessments, emotional support, and holistic strategies to manage symptoms and promote overall well-being. Whether you seek medical advice, nutritional guidance, mental health support, or alternative therapies, the diverse range of professionals available ensures that you can tailor your approach to menopause based on your unique needs and preferences. By collaborating with these professionals, you can navigate menopause with confidence, empowerment, and a comprehensive understanding of your health and well-being. Remember that seeking professional guidance is a proactive step toward embracing the transformative phase of menopause with grace and vitality.

Chapter Twelve

Glossary

Personal Stories

Menopause is a profound life transition that prompts women to explore various strategies for managing symptoms, promoting well-being, and embracing change. Many women choose to navigate this transformative phase through a natural approach, incorporating lifestyle changes, holistic practices, and self-care rituals. In this article, we'll delve into personal stories of women who have embraced a natural approach to menopause. Their experiences, insights, and journeys serve as a source of inspiration and guidance for those seeking to navigate menopause with authenticity, empowerment, and vitality.

•Anna's Journey: Embracing Mind-Body Connection

Anna, a 52-year-old woman, found herself in the midst of menopause with a desire to approach this phase holistically. She had heard about the benefits of mind-body practices, so she decided to explore yoga and meditation. Anna's journey was transformative – yoga helped her improve flexibility and joint health, while meditation provided a sense of calm that eased her emotional fluctuations. She shared, "Connecting with my body and breath through yoga has given me a newfound sense of strength. Meditation helps me stay centered amidst the challenges that come with menopause."

Anna also incorporated mindfulness into her daily routine. She practiced mindful eating, savoring each bite and tuning into her body's hunger cues. This approach to eating not only supported her physical well-being but also helped her cultivate a positive relationship with her body during this transition.

•Linda's Story: Nourishing Through Nutrition

Linda, at 50, decided to focus on nutrition as a cornerstone of her natural approach to menopause. She began researching foods that could support hormonal balance and alleviate symptoms. After consulting with a nutritionist, Linda revamped her diet to include more plant-based foods, fiber-rich grains, and nutrient-dense fruits and vegetables. She also embraced healthy fats, such as avocados and nuts, which are essential for hormone production.

Through her dietary changes, Linda experienced a reduction in hot flashes and increased energy levels. She shared, "Changing my diet was a game-changer. I felt like I was nurturing my body from the inside out. The natural approach empowered me to take control of my health during this transformative phase."

•Grace's Experience: Herbal Support and Holistic Healing

Grace, aged 48, turned to herbal remedies and holistic healing modalities to navigate menopause. She sought guidance from a naturopathic doctor who introduced her to adaptogenic herbs like ashwagandha and maca. These herbs supported her adrenal health and helped manage stress, which in turn alleviated some of her menopause-related symptoms.

Grace also explored acupuncture to address specific concerns like insomnia and mood swings. Regular acupuncture sessions not only provided relief but also fostered a sense of emotional balance and well-being. She shared, "Exploring natural remedies and holistic therapies allowed me to take an active role in my health. I've learned to listen to my body's cues and respond with gentleness and care."

•Samantha's Empowerment: Mindful Movement and Fitness

At 45, Samantha was determined to embrace menopause with a sense of empowerment. She discovered the power of mindful movement through dance and fitness. Samantha joined a dance class specifically designed for women in menopause, which combined cardiovascular exercise with mindful movement and stretching. This not only helped her maintain physical fitness but also uplifted her spirits and provided an outlet for self-expression.

Samantha also incorporated strength training into her routine to support her bone health. She shared, "Engaging in mindful movement has made me feel vibrant and alive. It's about celebrating what my body can do rather than focusing on limitations. Menopause became a journey of self-discovery and strength."

•Ella's Holistic Harmony: Balancing Body and Mind

Ella, aged 49, took a holistic approach to menopause by addressing both her physical and emotional well-being. She found solace in aromatherapy, using essential oils like lavender and chamomile to soothe stress and promote relaxation. These scents became a part of her daily rituals, contributing to her emotional equilibrium.

Ella also explored journaling as a way to process her feelings and experiences. Through writing, she connected with her inner thoughts and gained insights into her journey. "Holistic practices allowed me to create harmony within myself. The combination of aromatherapy, journaling, and other self-care rituals nurtured my mind, body, and soul."

Personal stories of women navigating menopause with a natural approach reflect the diversity of strategies and experiences that can shape this transformative phase. From embracing mind-body

practices like yoga and meditation to prioritizing nutrition, herbal support, fitness, and holistic healing, these women have discovered paths that align with their unique needs and desires. Their journeys underscore the power of listening to one's body, cultivating self-awareness, and choosing strategies that promote well-being and empowerment.

As these stories demonstrate, the natural approach to menopause is not a one-size-fits-all solution but rather a journey of exploration and self-discovery. Each woman's path is a testament to her strength, resilience, and willingness to embrace change with grace. By sharing these personal narratives, we celebrate the diverse ways in which women navigate menopause, inspiring others to embark on their own journeys with authenticity, empowerment, and vitality.

Key Terms and Concepts Explained

Understanding the key terms and concepts associated with menopause is essential for navigating this phase with knowledge and confidence. In this article, we'll explore and explain some of the crucial terms and concepts related to menopause, from hormonal changes to symptoms and treatment options.

1. Menopause:

- Explanation: Menopause is the natural biological process that marks the end of a woman's menstrual cycles and fertility. It is defined as the absence of menstruation for 12 consecutive months.

2. Perimenopause:

- Explanation: Perimenopause refers to the transitional period leading up to menopause. During this time, hormonal fluctuations can lead to irregular periods, changes in fertility, and the onset of menopausal symptoms.

3. Hormones:

- Explanation: Hormones are chemical messengers produced by the endocrine glands that regulate various bodily functions. During menopause, the levels of estrogen and progesterone decline, leading to physiological changes and symptoms.

4. Estrogen:

- Explanation: Estrogen is a primary female sex hormone produced primarily by the ovaries. It plays a crucial role in regulating the menstrual cycle, maintaining bone health, and supporting various bodily functions.

5. Progesterone:

- Explanation: Progesterone is another female sex hormone produced by the ovaries. It helps prepare the uterus for pregnancy and contributes to the regulation of the menstrual cycle.

6. Hot Flashes:

- Explanation: Hot flashes are sudden and intense sensations of heat that typically affect the face, neck, and chest. They are often accompanied by flushing and sweating and are a common menopausal symptom.

7. Night Sweats:

- Explanation: Night sweats are episodes of excessive sweating that occur during sleep. They are a nocturnal variation of hot flashes and can disrupt sleep and overall comfort.

8. Vaginal Dryness:

- Explanation: Vaginal dryness refers to a lack of moisture and lubrication in the vaginal area. It can lead to discomfort, pain during intercourse, and an increased risk of infections.

9. Osteoporosis:

- Explanation: Osteoporosis is a condition characterized by weakened bones that are more prone to fractures. During menopause, the decline in estrogen levels can contribute to bone loss and an increased risk of osteoporosis.

10. Hormone Replacement Therapy (HRT):

- Explanation: HRT involves the use of medications that contain hormones, such as estrogen and progesterone, to alleviate menopausal symptoms. It can be administered in various forms, including pills, patches, creams, and more.

11. Phytoestrogens:

- Explanation: Phytoestrogens are naturally occurring compounds found in plants that have a similar structure to estrogen. They can exert mild estrogenic effects in the body and may help alleviate some menopausal symptoms.

12. Mood Swings:

- Explanation: Mood swings are sudden and intense shifts in mood, often characterized by feelings of irritability, sadness, or anxiety. Hormonal changes during menopause can contribute to mood fluctuations.

13. Self-Care:

- Explanation: Self-care refers to intentional actions and practices that individuals engage in to promote their physical, emotional, and mental well-being. During menopause, self-care can include activities that alleviate symptoms and support overall health.

14. Mind-Body Practices:

- Explanation: Mind-body practices are techniques that emphasize the connection between the mind and the body. Examples include meditation, yoga, tai chi, and deep breathing, which can help manage stress and improve emotional well-being during menopause.

15. Holistic Approach:

- Explanation: A holistic approach involves considering the interconnectedness of various aspects of health, including physical, emotional, mental, and spiritual well-being. It involves addressing the whole person rather than isolated symptoms or issues.

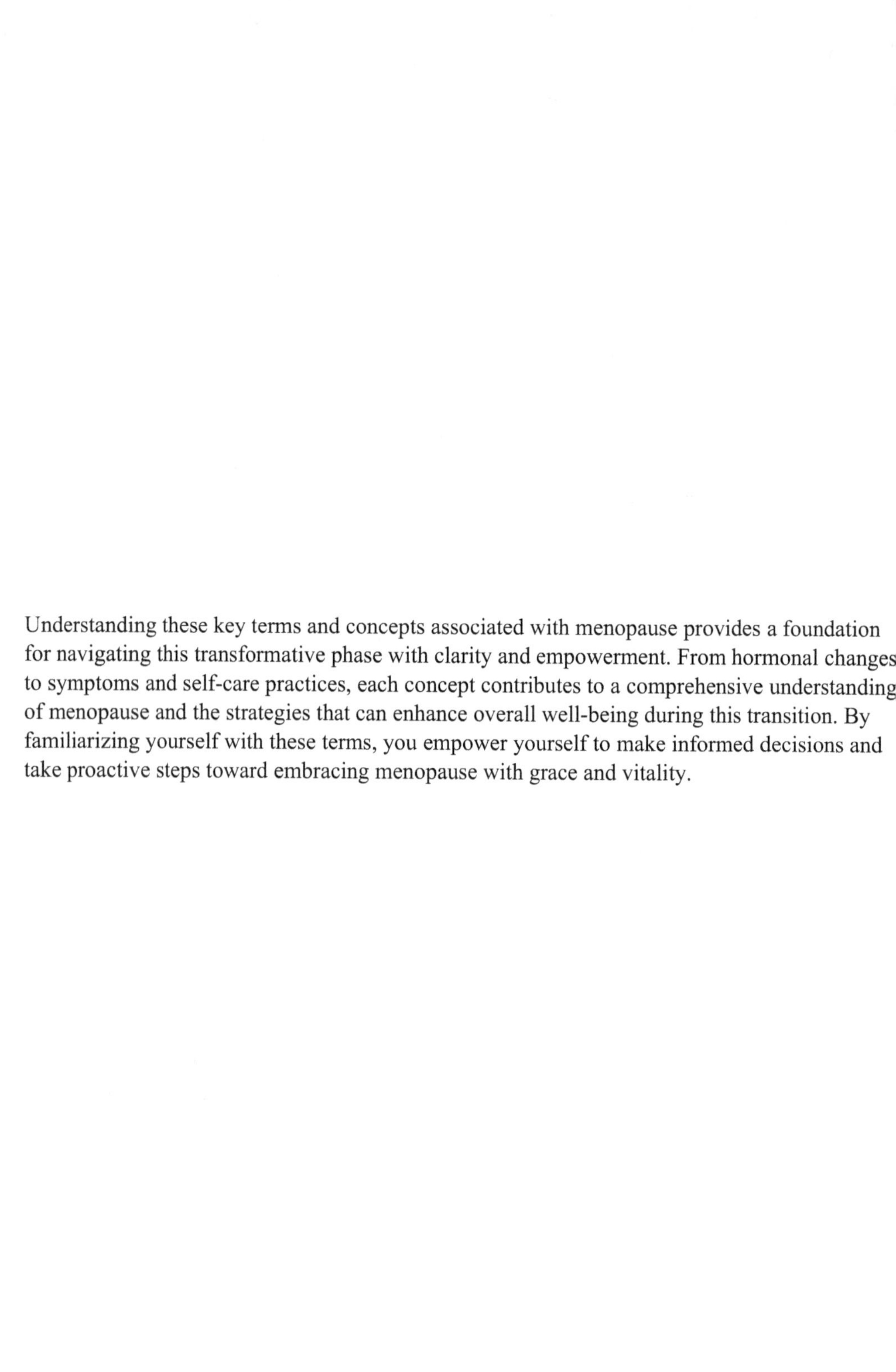

Understanding these key terms and concepts associated with menopause provides a foundation for navigating this transformative phase with clarity and empowerment. From hormonal changes to symptoms and self-care practices, each concept contributes to a comprehensive understanding of menopause and the strategies that can enhance overall well-being during this transition. By familiarizing yourself with these terms, you empower yourself to make informed decisions and take proactive steps toward embracing menopause with grace and vitality.